DIPLOMA IN PHARMACY

Pharmaceutical Chemistry I

Theory and Practical

Prof VN Rajasekaran

Formerly
Joint Director of Medical Education (Pharmacy)
Tamil Nadu
and
Professor of Pharmaceutical Chemistry
Madras Medical College, Chennai
and
Madurai Medical College, Madurai

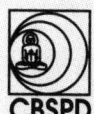

CBSPD

CBS Publishers & Distributors Pvt Ltd

New Delhi • Bengaluru • Chennai • Kochi • Kolkata • Lucknow • Mumbai
Hyderabad • Jharkhand • Nagpur • Patna • Pune • Uttarakhand

DIPLOMA IN PHARMACY

Pharmaceutical Chemistry I

Theory and Practical

ISBN: 978-93-85915-80-2

Copyright © Author and Publisher

CBS Edition: 2016

Reprint: 2017, 2018, 2019, 2020, 2021, 2023

Published by Satish Kumar Jain and Produced by Varun Jain for

CBS Publishers & Distributors Pvt Ltd

4819/XI Prahlad Street, 24 Ansari Road, Daryaganj, New Delhi 110 002, India.
Ph: 011-23289259, 23266861, 23266867 Fax: 011-23243014   Website: www.cbspd.com
                                                            e-mail: delhi@cbspd.com; cbspubs@airtelmail.in.
Corporate Office: 204 FIE, Industrial Area, Patparganj, Delhi 110 092
Ph: 011-4934 4934   Fax: 011-4934 4935   e-mail: publishing@cbspd.com; publicity@cbspd.com

Branches

*   **Bengaluru:** Seema House 2975, 17th Cross, KR Road, Banasankari 2nd Stage, Bengaluru
    560 070, Karnataka, India
    Ph: +91-80-26771678/79   Fax: +91-80-26771680   e-mail: bangalore@cbspd.com
*   **Chennai:** 7, Subbaraya Street, Shenoy Nagar, Chennai 600 030, Tamil Nadu, India
    Ph: +91-44-26680620, 26681266   Fax: +91-44-42032115   e-mail: chennai@cbspd.com
*   **Kochi:** 42/1325, 1326, Power House Road, Opp KSEB, Power House, Ernakulam 682 018, Kerala, India
    Ph: +91-484-4059061-65/67   Fax: +91-484-4059065   e-mail: kochi@cbspd.com
*   **Kolkata:** 147, Hind Ceramics Compound, 1st Floor, Nilgunj Road, Belghoria,
    Kolkata 700 056, West Bengal, India
    Ph: +033-25633055, 033-25633056   e-mail: kolkata@cbspd.com
*   **Lucknow:** Basement, Khushnuma Complex, 7-Meerabai Marg (Behind Jawahar Bhawan),
    Lucknow 226 001, UP, India
    Ph: 0522-4000032   e-mail: tiwari.lucknow@cbspd.com
*   **Mumbai:** PWD Shed. Gala no. 25/26, Ramchandra Bhatt Marg, Next to JJ Hospital Gate no. 2,
    Opp. Union Bank of India, Noorbaug, Mumbai 400 009, Maharashtra, India
    Ph: 022-66661880/89   Mob: 0-8424005858   e-mail: mumbai@cbspd.com

Representatives

• **Hyderabad**	0-9885175004	• **Jharkhand**	0-9811541605	• **Nagpur**	0-9421945513
• **Patna**	0-9334159340	• **Pune**	0-9623451994	• **Uttarakhand**	0-9716462459

Printed at SRK Graphics, Delhi, India

PREFACE

The E.R. '91 has come to stay and it is understood that even the few states which have not fallen in line due to various reasons have decided to do so from the academic year 1994 – '95. Hence it has become imperative that a new text book complying with the syllabus as prescribed for 'Pharmaceutical Chemistry - I' should be prepared . The immense popularity which the previous text book under E.R. 81 enjoyed amongst the students and the teaching fraternity has made it obligatory on my part to prepare a text book for the subject under E.R. 91 also.

It should be noted that the new syllabus has discarded the system of study of inorganic drugs based on chemical classification in favour of pharmacological classification. Even though this lays more stress on pharmacology than on the chemistry of the drugs, the treatment of the subject in this book is such that good emphasis is laid on the chemistry also to the extent necessary since almost all the drugs are chemicals only. A knowledge of their chemical properties will help to understand the rationale behind the tests for identity and also the storage conditions prescribed.

As in the earlier book, In this book also, the treatment of the subject is confined only to the bare essentials required in the syllabus and nothing more so as to present the students at the bottom level in pharmacy education a text book catering fully to their needs. Both theory and practical are included for the convenience of the teacher and the taught. All the standards, limit tests, assays etc. given in this book conform to I.P. 1985 only. Otherwise where the inorganic drug is not official in I.P. 1985, the standards in B.P. 1988 or I.P. 1966 as the case may be (where the drug has a monograph) have been adopted in theory and practical. Wherever it is simply mentioned as I.P., it means I.P. 1985. Similarly B.P. denotes B.P. 1988.

I trust and hope that the book will be of immense service to those for whom it is intended, viz. the Diploma in Pharmacy students.

V.N. RAJASEKARAN

III

PHARMACEUTICAL CHEMISTRY - I
THEORY (75 hours)

1. General discussion of the following inorganic compounds including physical and chemical properties, medicinal and pharmaceutical uses, storage conditions and chemical incompatibility.

   (A) Acids, bases and buffers – Boric acid*, Hydrochloric acid, Strong ammonium hydroxide, Calcium hydroxide, Sodium hydroxide and official buffers.

   (B) Antioxidants – Hypophosphorous acid, Sulphur dioxide, Sodium bisulphite, Sodium metabisulphite. Sodium thiosulphate, Nitrogen and Sodium nitrite.

   (C) Gastrointestinal agents :-

      (i) Acidifying agents – Dilute hydrochloric acid:

      (ii) Antacids – Sodium bicarbonate, Aluminium hydroxide gel, Aluminium phosphate, Calcium carbonate, Magnesium carbonate, Magnesium trisilicate, Magnesium oxide, Combinations of antacid preparations.

      (iii) Protectives and adsorbents – Bismuth subcarbonate and Kaolin.

      (iv) Saline Cathartics – Sodium potassium tartrate and Magnesium sulphate.

   (D) Topical agents

      (i) Protectives – Talc, Zinc oxide, Calamine, Zinc stearate, Titanium dioxide, Silicone polymers.

      (ii) Antimicrobiais and Astringents – Hydrogen peroxide*, Potassium permanganate, Chlorinated lime, Iodine, Solutions of iodine, Povidone-iodine, Boric acid, Borax,

Silver nitrate, Mild silver protein, Mercury, Yellow mercuric oxide, Ammoniated mercury.

(iii) Sulphur and its compounds - Sublimed sulphur, Precipitated sulphur, Selenium sulphide.

(iv) Astringents - Alum and Zinc sulphate.

(E) Dental products – Sodium fluoride, Stannous fluoride. Sodium metaphosphate, Strontium chloride, Zinc chloride.

(F) Inhalants – Oxygen, Carbon dioxide, Nitrous oxide.

(G) Respiratory stimulants – Ammonium carbonate.

(H) Expectorants and Emetics – Ammonium chloride, Potassium iodide, Antimony potassium tartrate.

(I) Antidotes - Sodium nitrite.

2. Major Intra and Extracellular Electrolytes –

(A) Electrolytes used for replacement therapy – Sodium chloride and its preparations, Potassium chloride and its preparations.

(B) Physiological acid – base balance and electrolytes used – Sodium acetate, Potassium acetate, Sodium bicarbonate injection, Sodium citrate, Potassium citrate, Sodium lactate injection. Ammonium chloride and its injection.

(C) Combination of oral electrolyte powders and solutions.

3. Inorganic official compounds of Iron, Iodine and Calcium, Ferrous sulphate and Calcium gluconate.

4. Radio pharmaceuticals and contrast media – Radioactivity, Alpha, Beta and Gamma radiations, Biological effects of radiations, Measurement of radioactivity, G.M. counter, Radio isotopes – Their uses, storage and precautions with special reference to the official preparations.

Radio opaque contrast media - Barium sulphate.

5. Quality control of Drugs and Pharmaceuticals - Importance of quality control, significant errors, methods used for quality control, sources of impurities in pharmaceuticals, limit tests for arsenic, chloride, sulphate, iron and heavy metals.

6. Identification tests for cations and anions as per Indian Pharmacopoeia.

PRACTICAL (75 hours)

1. Identification tests for inorganic compounds particularly drugs and pharmaceuticals.

2. Limit tests for chloride, sulphate, arsenic, iron and heavy metals.

3. Assay of inorganic pharmaceuticals involving each of the following compounds marked with (*) under theory.

   (a) Acid-base titrations (at least 3).

   (b) Redox titrations (one each of permanganimetry and iodimetry).

   (c) Precipitation titrations (at least 3).

   (d) Complexometric titrations (calcium and magnesium).

CONTENTS

X

SECTION B - PRACTICAL

CHAPTER		Page

SOLUBILITY DESCRIPTIONS

The solubility descriptions in this book denote the following ranges :

Description	Approximate quantities of solvent by volume required to dissolve 1 part of solute by weight.
Very soluble	Less than 1 part
Freely soluble	From 1 to 10 parts
Soluble	From 10 to 30 parts
Sparingly soluble	From 30 to 100 parts
Slightly soluble	From 100 to 1,000 parts
Very slightly soluble	From 1,000 to 10,000 parts
Practically insoluble	More than 10,000 parts

Section A
THEORY

CHAPTER 1

ACIDITY, BASICITY, pH AND BUFFERS

The acidity and alkalinity of a solution may be found out by measuring the concentrations of hydrogen and hydroxyl ions respectively in gram equivalents per litre. These concentrations may be expressed as pH and pOH as given below:

$$pH = \log_{10} \frac{1}{[H^+]} = -\log_{10}[H^+]$$

$$pOH = \log_{10} \frac{1}{[OH^-]} = -\log_{10}[OH^-]$$

where $[H^+]$ and $[OH^-]$ represent the concentrations of hydrogen and hydroxyl ions respectively in gram equivalents per litre.

Even the most highly purified water possesses a small but definite conductivity due to ionisation to a small extent :

$$2H_2O \rightleftharpoons H_3O^+ + OH^-$$

The hydrogen ion remains in water as the hydronium or the hydroxonium ion H_3O^+ but for the sake of simplicity the following more familiar equation is used :

$$H_2O \rightleftharpoons H^+ + OH^-$$

If we apply the law of mass action to this equation, we obtain,

$$\frac{[H^+][OH^-]}{[H_2O]} = \text{a constant } K$$

where $[H^+]$, $[OH^-]$ and $[H_2O]$ are the concentrations of the hydrogen ion, hydroxyl ion and undissociated water respectively.

In pure water $[H_2O]$ is a constant Therefore $[H^+][OH^-] = Kw$ where Kw is known as the ionic product of water. This is the product got by multiplying the concentrations of the hydrogen and hydroxyl ions.

It has been determined that the experimental value of Kw is 1×10^{-14} gram ions per litre. Therefore in pure water or in a neutral solution, the concentrations of hydrogen ions and hydroxyl ions are equal. So $[H^+] = [OH^-] = \sqrt{Kw} = 10^{-7}$ gram ions per litre at 25°C. The hydrogen ion concentration gives the acidity of a solution and the hydroxyl ion concentration gives the alkalinity of a solution.

However this quantity is very small and inconvenient for usage. Therefore another practicable method has been devised to express the hydrogen and hydroxyl ion concentrations. As per this method, the hydrogen ion concentration, the hydroxyl ion concentration and the ionic product of water are converted first to their reciprocals as given below:

$$\frac{1}{[H^+]} \times \frac{1}{[OH^-]} = \frac{1}{Kw}$$

The reciprocals are then converted into their logarithms and are respectively termed as pH, pOH and pKw.

pH + pOH = pKw

or 7 + 7 = 14 in the case of pure water.

Since pH and pOH values are complementary to each other, the pH notation only is conveniently used to express both acidity and alkalinity. Thus a solution having a pH value of 7 is neutral. Any solution having a pH value below 7 is acid. The lower the pH value, the higher is the acidity of the solution. Thus a solution with a pH value of 2 is more acid than a solution with a pH value of 5. A pH value above 7 denotes that the solution is alkaline. However the more the pH value the higher is the alkalinity of the solution. Thus a solution having a pH value of 12 is more alkaline than one having a pH value of say 9.

ACIDS AND BASES

According to modern concepts, an acid is a substance which can donate a proton. A base is a substance which can combine with a proton. A proton here means the hydrogen ion since the hydrogen atom contains a proton in the nucleus with an extra nuclear electron. With the loss of the electron, the hydrogen atom with only the single proton in the nucleus becomes the hydrogen ion.

The acids can be divided into mineral acids and organic acids. Examples of mineral acids are perchloric acid ($HClO_4$), sulphuric acid (H_2SO_4), hydrochloric acid (HCl), hydriodic acid (HI), nitric acid (HNO_3) etc. Examples of organic acids are formic acid, acetic acid, tartaric acid, citric acid etc. Examples of bases are ammonia, sodium hydroxide, potassium hydroxide, tetraethyl or tetrabutyl ammonium hydroxide etc.

BUFFERS

Th pH of a solution, even when carefully adjusted, may not remain the same for long due to some extraneous factors. For example if the containers are made from cheap glass, the glass may release alkali into the solution and because of this the pH of the solution rises. The pH change may also be brought about by CO_2, Cl_2 or ammonia from the atmosphere. Because of this the medicament in the solution may undergo decomposition. Also it is necessary that solutions of certain medicaments like thiamine (stable at a pH between 2.5 and 4.5), ascorbic acid (stable at a pH between 5.5 and 7) and cyanocobalamin (stable at a pH between 3.6 and 5.5), hormones like insulin (stable at a pH of 3) and oxytocin (stable at a pH between 2.5 and 4.5) and several alkaloids, antibiotics etc. should be kept at a definite pH to promote the stability of these medicaments in solution. For this purpose *buffers* are added to the solutions.

A buffer solution will prevent any change in pH in the solution to which it is added when small quantities of acids or bases are added. A buffer solution or a buffer is a solution containing a weak acid and its salt with a strong base (acid buffer) and a weak base and its salt with a strong acid (basic buffer). Let us take the example of an acid buffer consisting of acetic acid and sodium acetate ($CH_3COOH + CH_3COONa$), a typical combination of a weak acid and its salt. The buffering mechanism of this solution or in other words how it resists any change in pH in the solution to which it is added can be explained as below:

3

1. When a small quantity of an acid is added to this solution, the acetate anions derived from the almost complete dissociation of sodium acetate combine with the hydrogen ions of the added acid to produce relatively undissociated acetic acid :

$$CH_3COONa \rightleftharpoons CH_3COO^- + Na^+$$

$$HCl \rightleftharpoons H^+ + Cl^-$$

$$CH_3COO^- + H^+ \rightleftharpoons CH_3COOH$$

Acetic acid
(weakly ionised)

2. Similarly when a small quantity of a base is added to the solution, the hydroxyl ions from the base are neutralised by the hydrogen ions from the acetic acid in the buffer solution to form practically undissociated water.

$$CH_3COOH \rightleftharpoons CH_3COO^- + H^+$$

$$NaOH \rightleftharpoons Na^+ + OH^-$$

$$H^+ + OH^- \rightleftharpoons H_2O$$

Thus as per the buffer capacity of the buffer solution, any change in the pH of the solution to which the buffer solution has been added is prevented and this helps in maintaining the pH of the solution at the same level for long periods.

OFFICIAL BUFFER SOLUTIONS

There are various methods for preparing buffer solutions. The standard buffer solutions given in the I.P. 1985 are prepared by mixing 0.2 N solution of hydrochloric acid or 0.2 N sodium hydroxide solution with definite quantities of 0.2 M solutions of certain substances such as potassium hydrogen phthalate or potasium chloride etc. For example the *hydrochloric acid buffers* from pH range 1.2 to 2.2 are prepared by mixing 50 ml of 0.2 M potassium chloride solution with specified quantities of 0.2 N hydrochloric acid in a 200 ml volumetric flask, diluting to the mark and mixing. Similarly the *acid phthalate buffers*

4

from pH range 2.2 to 4 are prepared by mixing 50 ml of potassium hydrogen phthalate solution and specified quantities of 0.2N hydrochloric acid in a 200 ml volumetric flask using the same procedure. *The neutralised phthalate buffers* from pH range 4.2 to 5.8 are prepared by mixing 50 ml of potasium hydrogen phthalate solution with specified volumes of sodium hydroxide solution. The *phosphate buffers* from pH 5.8 to 8.0 are prepared by mixing 50 ml of potassium hydrogen phosphate solution with specified volumes of sodium hydroxide solution. Finally the *alkaline borate buffers* from pH 8 to 10 are prepared by mixing 50 ml of boric acid and potassium chloride solution with specified volumes of sodium hydroxide solution. Using these buffer solutions it is possible to adjust any solution of a medicament to the desired pH.

These standard buffer solutions are solutions of standard pH. They can be used for reference purposes in the measurement of pH and also for doing any tests where adjustment to a definite pH is required. Certain precautions are given in I.P. for preparing these buffer solutions. All the solid reagents except boric acid should be dried at $110^{\circ}C - 120^{\circ}C$ for one hour before use. Freshly boiled and cooled water only should be used for preparing these solutions. This is water free from carbon dioxide which, if present, may affect the pH. All the solutions should be stored in containers made of chemically resistant alkali-free glass and used within three months of their preparation. Any solution which has turned cloudy and or has deteriorated in any other way should not be used. The methods of preparation of the basic solutions that is hydrochloric acid, 0.2 N, sodium hydroxide, 0.2 N, potassium hydrogen phthalate 0.2 M, potassium dihydrogen phosphate 0.2 M, boric acid and potassium chloride, 0.2 M and potassium chloride, 0.2 M are given in detail in the I.P. which should be strictly followed.

CHAPTER 2

CHEMISTRY OF SOME ACIDS AND BASES OF MEDICINAL OR PHARMACEUTICAL IMPORTANCE

1. BORIC ACID, H_3BO_3

Preparation: Boric acid occurs in volcanic jets of steam. The steam is condensed and cooled. Crude boric acid crystallizes out. It is purified by recrystallization.

Native borates may also be decomposed with a mineral acid.

$$Na_2B_4O_7 + H_2SO_4 + 5H_2O \longrightarrow Na_2SO_4 + 4H_3BO_3$$

The boric acid is allowed to crystallize after filtration. It is collected by filtration, washed free from soluble sulphate and dried.

Physical and Chemical Properties: Boric acid occurs in three forms.

(1) Transparent, smooth, pearly scales.
(2) Triclinic crystals and
(3) a white bulky powder.

These forms are stable in air. The scale and crystalline forms can be used for preparing solutions. The powder can be used in dusting powders and ointments.

Boric acid is soluble 1 in 25 in water and in 4 parts of glycerol. It volatilizes appreciably from aqueous solutions at 60^0C and above.

Orthoboric acid is a weak acid. It is a tribasic acid and cannot be titrated with standard alkali directly. However when mixed with glycerol or mannitol, a stronger monobasic acid is formed which can be titrated with alkali directly (refer assay) using phenolphthalein as indicator.Orthoboric acid turns litmus a dull claret red. Only the alkali borates such as sodium borate or borax are soluble in water. Their solutions have a strong basic reaction.

6

When orthoboric acid is heated at 100°C or slightly above, it is converted to metaboric acid by loss of a molecule of water:

$$H_3BO_3 \xrightarrow[100°C]{\Delta} HBO_2 + H_2O$$
$$\text{Metaboric acid}$$

Further heating to approximately 160°C results in the formation of tetraboric acid called as pyroboric acid:

$$4HBO_2 \xrightarrow{\Delta} H_2B_4O_7 + H_2O$$
$$\text{Pyroboric acid}$$

Still further heating converts the residue to boron trioxide, a glass-like solid:

$$H_2B_4O_7 \xrightarrow{\Delta} 2B_2O_3 + H_2O$$

Boron trioxide dissolves in water to form orthoboric acid:

$$3H_2O + B_2O_3 \longrightarrow 2H_3BO_3$$

The borates are salts of neither H_3BO_3 or HBO_2 but mainly of $H_2B_4O_7$. A solution of boric acid in water contains only a minute amount of $H_2B_4O_7$ but when neutralised with a base and concentrated, the more crystalline salt $Na_2B_4O_7$ will form.

It is official in I.P.

Official Tests for Identity

1. Dissolve the sample in a mixture of methyl alcohol and concentrated sulphuric acid. Ignite the solution. The flame burns with a green border. This is due to the formation of methyl borate.

2. Dissolve the sample in boiling water and cool. The solution is faintly acid.

Non-official Tests for Identity

1. Acidify a 5 per cent w/v solution with hydrochoric acid, moisten a piece of turmeric paper with this solution and dry.The colour of the paper becomes pink or brownish red.

7

Pour dilute ammonia solution or solution of sodium hydroxide on the paper: The colour changes to blue or greenish black.

2. Ignite in porcelain dish a solution in alcohol. It burns and the flame is tinged green. This is due to the formation of volatile ethyl borate.

Standard: Contains between 99.5 per cent and 100.5 per cent of H_3BO_3 calculated with reference to the substance dried over sulphuric acid for five hours.

Storage condition: The substance is quite stable in air. So there is no special storage condition other than the following:

Store in a well closed container.

Chemical Incompatibility: Boric acid is always externally used as a local anti-infective either alone or in combination with other substances such as zinc oxide, starch etc. Since it is a weak acid, it does not affect the other substances. However if glycerin or any other polyhydric alcohol is present, it is converted to a stronger monobasic acid which may react with any base present.

Assay: An accurately weighed quantity of the sample is dissolved in a mixture of water and glycerol previosly neutralised to phenolphthalin and titrated with N/1 sodium hydroxide using phenolphthalein as indicator. A permanent pale pink colour is the end point.

As already stated since boric acid is a weak acid, it cannot be titrated with alkali directly. Glycerol combines with boric acid to form a monobasic acid known as glyceryl boric acid which is strong enough to be directly titrated with N/1 sodium hydroxide and give a satisfactory end point:

Glycerol   Boric acid   Glyceryl boric acid

Polyhydric alcohols such as glycols and mannitol produce a similar result:

$$
\begin{array}{c}
CH_2OH \\
|\\
(HO-C-H)_2 \\
|\\
2\ H-C-OH \quad HO \\
\qquad + \qquad \diagdown \\
\qquad\qquad B-OH\rightarrow \\
\qquad / \\
H-C-OH \quad HO \\
|\\
CH_2OH
\end{array}
\qquad
\begin{array}{c}
CH_2OH \qquad\qquad CH_2OH \\
|\qquad\qquad\qquad\quad |\\
(HO-C-H)_2 \quad (H-C-OH)_2 \\
|\qquad\qquad\qquad\quad |\\
H-C-O \qquad\quad O-C-H \\
\quad\diagdown \qquad / \\
\qquad B \\
\quad / \qquad \diagdown \\
H-C-O \qquad\quad O-C-H \\
|\qquad\qquad\qquad\quad |\\
CH_2OH \qquad\qquad CH_2OH
\end{array}
$$

Mannitol   Mannityl boric acid

Medicinal or Pharmaceutical Use: Pharmaceutical aid and local anti- infective.

2. HYDROCHLORIC ACID, HCl

Hydrochloric acid is prepared by dissolving hydrogen chloride gas in water.

Preparation of Hydrogen Chloride.

1. Hydrogen chloride may be made by reacting sodium chloride (common salt) with sulphuric acid. The reaction takes place in two steps.

$$NaCl + H_2SO_4 \longrightarrow NaHSO_4 + HCl$$
Sodium bisulphate

$$NaHSO_4 + NaCl \longrightarrow Na_2SO_4 + HCl$$
Sodium sulphate
(salt cake)

The hydrogen chloride in the first step above known as the 'pan acid' is comparatively more pure whereas the hydrogen chloride obtained in the second step along with the salt cake is less pure and is known as 'muriatic acid' of commerce. Muriatic acid is a yellow liquid.

2. In this method the hydrogen and chlorine obtained in the electrolysis of sodium chloride in the manufacture of caustic soda are burned preferably using quartz bunsen burners.

$$H_2 + Cl_2 \longrightarrow 2\,HCl$$

100% pure hydrogen chloride is formed in this method.

Physical and Chemical Properties.

Hydrogen chloride is a colourless gas with an acrid irritating odour and an acid taste. It is heavier than air and is very soluble in water. About 460 ml of the gas dissolve in 1 ml of water at at $20^{\circ}C$ at 760 mm pressure.

Hydrochloric Acid, I.P. is an aqueous solution of hydrogen chloride in water. It contains between 35 per cent and 38 per cent w/w of HCl. It is a clear, colourless, fuming liquid with a pungent taste.

Hydrochloric acid combines directly with alkalis such as ammonia and sodium hydroxide. These are known as neutralization reactions.

$$NH_3 + HCl \longrightarrow NH_4Cl$$

$$NaOH + HCl \longrightarrow NaCl + H_2O$$

It also reacts with metals to form the corresponding chlorides.

$$2Na + 2HCl \longrightarrow 2NaCl + H_2\uparrow$$

It releases carbon dioxide from carbonates and bicarbonates.

$$Na_2CO_3 + 2HCl \longrightarrow 2\,NaCl + H_2CO_3$$
$$\text{Carbonic acid}$$

$$H_2CO_3 \longrightarrow H_2O + CO_2\uparrow$$

$$NaHCO_3 + HCl \longrightarrow NaCl + CO_2\uparrow + H_2O$$

This is another type of neutralisation reaction. It gives a curdy white percipitate with silver nitrate.

$$AgNO_3 + HCl \longrightarrow AgCl\downarrow + HNO_3$$

The silver chloride precipitate is photosensitive and becomes slightly pink on exposure to light. It is very sparingly soluble in water.

Hydrochloric acid produces sulphur dioxide on reaction with a sulphite.

$$Na_2SO_3 + 2HCl \longrightarrow 2\,NaCl + H_2SO_3$$
$$\text{Sulphurous acid}$$

$$H_2SO_3 \longrightarrow SO_2\uparrow + H_2O$$

It produces hydrogen sulphide with sodium sulphide and decomposes sodium thiosulphate to precipitate sulphur.

$$Na_2S + 2HCl \longrightarrow 2\,NaCl + H_2S\uparrow$$
$$Na_2S_2O_3 + 2HCl \longrightarrow 2NaCl + SO_2\uparrow + S\downarrow + H_2O$$

It is official in I.P.

Official Tests for Identity

1. When a sample is neutralised and diluted with water, it gives the reactions of chlorides (see Chapter 13).

2. When the sample is added to pot. permanganate, chlorine is evolved.

Non-official Tests for Identity

1. When the sample is added to silver nitrate solution, a white, curdy precipitate of silver chloride is formed. It is insoluble in nitric acid but soluble in ammonia solution. In ammonia it forms the soluble diammino-silver chloride, Ag $(NH_3)_2Cl$.

2. It gives with ammonia thick white fumes (formation of ammonium chloride).

3. Chlorine is produced when hydrochloric acid is heated with manganese dioxide.

Standard: Hydrochloric Acid is an aqueous solution of hydrogen chloride gas (HCl) in water. It contains not less than 35% w/w and not more than 38% w/w of HCl.

Storage Condition: Hydrogen chloride gas volatilises from hydrochloric acid when exposed to atmosphere till a constant boiling mixture of 20.24% boiling at 110°C is formed. Therefore hydrochloric

11

acid should be stored in glass-stoppered containers securely closed at a temperature not exceeding 30°C.

Chemical Incompatibility: Since this is an acid, it is incompatible with all bases and alkalis. It will release carbon dioxide when it comes into contact with carbonates and bicarbonates and sulphur dioxide with sulphites. Sometimes hydrochloric acid is deliberately added to give an acid pH for the stability of the active ingredient. Also it may be added for dissolving some substances in water.For example quinine sulphate and quinine hydrochloride are converted into soluble quinine bisulphate and quinine dihydrochloride by adding dilute hydrochloric acid.

When hydrochloric acid is added to an emulsion containing an anionic emulsifying agent such as the sodium or potassium soap, the emulsifying agent is decomposed and the emulsion breaks up.

Assay: An accurately weighed quantity of the acid is diluted with water and titrated against N/1 sodium hydroxide using methyl orange solution as the indicator. End point is the appearance of a faint yellow colour.

Medicinal and Pharmaceutical Uses

Pharmaceutical aid (acidifying agent): Hydrochloric acid is used in cases of achlorhydria (lack of hydrochloric acid in the gastric juice) in the form of Dilute Hydrochloric Acid, I.P.

It is also used in the manufacture of glucose form corn starch, for extracting glue (gelatin) from bones and as a reagent in the laboratory.

3. STRONG AMMONIA SOLUTION

Strong ammonia solution is prepared by dissolving ammonia gas in water.

Preparation:

(a) Previously ammonia was obtained as a bye-product of the production of coal gas. This ammoniacal gas liquor is a brown unpleasant-smelling tarry liquid and it contains both free ammonia and ammonium salts. When it is distilled with lime and the resulting ammonia gas is absorbed in sulphuric acid, ammonium sulphate which is used as a fertilizer is produced.

12

(b) Ammonia is made synthetically by the Haber process in which nitrogen and hydrogen are combined in the presence of a catalyst (iron and molybdenum) maintained at a temperature of 500°C under 200 atmospheres.

$$N_2 + 3H_2 \longrightarrow 2NH_3$$

Physical and Chemical Properties

Ammonia is a colourless gas having a strong, pungent, characteristic odour. It is about one-half as heavy as air. At 15°C, one millilitre of water of water dissolves 727 ml of the gas. Its solutions are lighter than water. All the gas may be expelled from its solutions by boiling. Ammonia exists in aqueous solution mainly in the form of NH_3 only. A small quantity reacts with water to form NH_4OH:

$$NH_3 + HOH \longrightarrow NH_4OH$$

Ammonium salts usually behave like alkali metal salts. However tv differences can be pointed out: (1) Ammonium salts are volatile (2 Ammonium salts are hydrolysed to a great extent in solution since the are derived from a comparatively weak base.

Strong Ammonia Solution is prepared by passing the gas from an of the sources mentioned under preparation into water till a weight pe ml of 0.900 to 0.915 g is obtained for the solution.

It neutralises acids to form salts (ammonium salts and water).

$$NH_4OH + HCl \longrightarrow NH_4Cl + H_2O$$

It reacts with some metallic salts and the metallic hydroxides are precipitated.

$$FeCl_3 + 3NH_4OH \longrightarrow Fe(OH)_3 + 3NH_4Cl$$
Ferric hydroxide
(Brown ppt)

$$ZnSO_4 + 2NH_4OH \longrightarrow Zn(OH)_2 + (NH_4)_2SO_4$$
Zinc hydroxide
(White ppt)

Ammonia forms molecular complexes with certain metals such as silver and copper.

$$Ag^+ + 2NH_3 \rightleftharpoons [Ag(NH_3)_2]^+$$

$$Cu^{2+} + 4NH_3 \rightleftharpoons [Cu(NH_3)_4]^{2+}$$

The copper molecular complex, that is the ammoniacal solution of cupric hydroxide known as cuoxam is used as reagent for cellulose, that is for cotton which contains almost pure cellulose. Cellulose is soluble in cuoxam.

Strong Ammonia Solution is official in B.P. '88 and also in I.P.'66 as Ammonia Solution Strong.

Tests for Identity
Official

1. Dilute freely with water. The solution produced is strongly alkaline (which may be tested with red litmus or any other suitable indicator).

2. Dip a glass rod in hydrochloric acid and keep it near the surface of the solution. Dense white fumes are produced (this is due to the formation of ammonium chloride).

Non-official

When Nessler's regeant (alkaline potassium mercuri-iodide solution) is added to Ammonia Solution Strong, a yellow to brown colour or precipitate is formed.

Standard: Contains not less than 27 per cent w/w and not more than 30 per cent w/w of NH_3.

Storage Condition: Since ammonia volatilises from solution at room temperature, Strong Ammonia Solution should be stored in a well-closed container at a temperature not exceeding 20°C.

Chemical Incompatibility

As ammonia is a base, it is incompatible with acids. It is also incompatible with salts of metals such as iron, zinc and copper precipitating their hydroxides. Alkaloidal salts like quinine hydrochloride or strychnine hydrochloride are decomposed by the

14

addition of ammonia and the insoluble free alkaloids are formed. However quinine is soluble where alcohol is also present along with ammonia.

Assay: An accurately weighed quantity of the solution is transferred to a conical flask containing a measured quantity of $N/1$ sulphuric acid. The excess of acid is back-titrated against $N/1$ sodium hydroxide using methyl red as indicator.

Medicinal and Pharmaceutical Uses: As a stimulant and restorative. It is also used as a reagent in the laboratory. Ammonia is also used in the production of nitric acid, soda ash, plastics, nylon, lacquers, resins, dyes and refrigerants. Liquid Ammonia is used as a refrigerant.

4. SODIUM HYDROXIDE (CAUSTIC SODA), NaOH
Preparation

(a) Chemical Method

This depends upon the interaction of sodium carbonate with calcium hydroxide to form sodium hydroxide and insoluble calcium carbonate.

$$Ca(OH)_2 + Na_2CO_3 \longrightarrow 2NaOH + CaCO_3\downarrow$$

(b) Electrolytic Method

Brine is eloectrolysed in an electrolytic cell with carbon anode and metallic cathode. The respective ions, sodium and chlorine, move to cathode and anode respectively. The following reactions take place:

$$NaCl \rightleftharpoons Na^+ + Cl^-$$

At the Anode   **At the Cathode**

$$Cl^- \longrightarrow Cl \qquad Na^+ \longrightarrow Na$$

$$Cl + Cl \longrightarrow Cl_2 \qquad 2Na + 2H_2O \longrightarrow 2NaOH + H_2$$

These two gases hydrogen and chlorine are collected separately or allowed to react to form hydrogen chloride.

$$H_2 + Cl_2 \longrightarrow 2HCl$$

15

Physical and Chemical Properties

(a) Physical Properties

Sodium hydroxide occurs in dry, hard, brittle, white or nearly white sticks, in fused masses, in small pellets, in flakes and in other forms. It is very deliquescent and rapidly absorbs moisture and carbon dioxide form the air. Sodium hydroxide is very caustic, damaging tissues.

Sodium hydroxide dissolves freely in water (1 in 1) with evolution of heat. It is soluble in alcohol, ether and glycerin.

(b) Chemical Properties

1. Since sodium hydroxide is so highly ionized when dissolved in water, it is one of the strongest bases. The basic properties are entirely due to the hydroxyl ion:

$$NaOH \longrightarrow Na^+ + OH^-$$

2. It reacts with acid to form salt and water.

$$NaOH + HCl \longrightarrow NaCl + H_2O$$

3. It absorbs carbon dioxide from the atmosphere or when passed through it to form sodium carbonate:

$$H_2O + CO_2 \rightleftarrows H_2CO_3$$

$$2NaOH + H_2CO_3 \longrightarrow Na_2CO_3 + 2H_2O$$

4. Sodium hydroxide reacts with the salts of all metals in solution precipitating all as their hydroxides except the hydroxides of alkali metals and ammonium.

$$NH_4Cl + NaOH \longrightarrow NH_4OH + NaCl$$

$$FeCl_3 + 3NaOH \longrightarrow Fe(OH)_3 + 3NaCl$$
Ferric chloride   Ferric hydroxide

In some cases, excess of sodium hydroxide will redissolve the precipitate.

$$AlCl_3 + 3NaOH \longrightarrow Al(OH)_3 + 3NaCl$$
Aluminium chloride   Aluminium hydroxide

$$Al(OH)_3 + NaOH \longrightarrow NaAlO_2 + 2H_2O$$
Sodium aluminate

5. Sodium hydroxide is used for saponifying fats and oils to form soap. The fat or oil is heated with the alkali solution and the soap formed is "salted out" by adding sodium chloride solution:

For Ex.	$CH_2O.OC.C_{17}H_{35}$ $CHO.OCC_{17}H_{35}$ $CH_2O.OC.C_{17}H_{35}$ Tristearin (a fat)	$+3\ NaOH \rightarrow$

$3C_{17}H_{35}COONa$ (soap)
\+
CH_2OH
$\mid$
$CHOH$
$\mid$
CH_2OH

Glycerol

It is official in I.P.

Official Tests for Identity

Dissolved in water, the solution gives the reactions of sodium (see Chapter 13).

Standard: Contains not less than 95 per cent of total alkali calculated as NaOH including not more than 3 per cent of Na_2CO_3.

Storage Condition: Since it absorbs moisture and carbon dioxide forming sodium carbonate, it should be stored in a well-closed container.

Chemical Incompatibility

Since it is a strong alkali, it is incompatible with acids. It is also incompatible with salts of certain metals such as iron, zinc and copper precipitating their hydroxides. Alkaloidal salts are decomposed by the addition of sodium hydroxide and free alkaloids are released.

Assay: Sodium hydroxide should contain at least 95 per cent of total alkali including not more than 3 per cent of sodium carbonate.

For estimating total alkali an accurately weighed quantity is dissolved in carbon dioxide-free water, cooled and titrated with N/1 sulphuric acid using phenolphthalein as indicator till the pink colour of the solution is discharged. Then methyl orange solution is added and the titration is continued till a persistent faint pink colour is obtained.

The total titre value is used for calculating total alkali (that is sodium hydroxide + sodium carbonate present) which is calculated as NaOH only. The amount of Na_2CO_3 present is calculated by taking the titre value obtained after adding methyl orange solution. This should not exceed 3 per cent and the total alkali should be not less than 95 per cent.

In this titration, the sodium hydroxide only reacts with acid when phenophthalein only is the indicator. After the end point is obtained indicated by the disappearance of the pink colour of the phenolphthalein, the sodium carbonate reacts with the acid.

$$2NaOH + H_2SO_4 \longrightarrow Na_2SO_4 + 2H_2O$$

$$Na_2CO_3 + H_2SO_4 \longrightarrow Na_2SO_4 + CO_2\uparrow + H_2O$$

Medicinal and Pharmaceutical Uses: Sodium hydroxide is so caustic that it finds little use in medicine. However it is used in the preparation of soap and as a pharmaceutical aid. It is also used as a reagent in the laboratory.

5. CALCIUM HYDROXIDE (SLAKED LIME), $Ca(OH)_2$

Preparation: Limestone (calcium carbonate) is heated to redness in kilns:

$$CaCO_3 \longrightarrow CaO + CO_2\uparrow$$

Limestone   Quick lime

The quick lime is slaked by adding water carefully. It crumbles to a powder giving rise to a lot of heat.

$$CaO + H_2O \longrightarrow Ca(OH)_2$$

The calcium hydroxide is mixed with excess of water which is allowed to settle. The supernatant liquid is decanted and the residue is dried in air.

Physical and Chemical Properties

Calcium hydroxide is a soft, white powder with an alkaline and slightly bitter taste. It is slightly soluble in water. A saturated solution contains about 1.7 g of calcium hydroxide in 1 litre of water, that is solubility is 0.17% w/v and the solubility is reduced when the solution is heated. The solubility can be increased to 26 g per litre or 2.6 per cent if the calcium hydroxie is dissolved in 10 per cent sucrose solution. The increased solubility is due to the formation of calcium sucrosate. Calcium hydroxide is insoluble in alcohol. Aqueous solution of calcium hydroxide is alkaline to phenolphthalein and other common indicators.

Calcium hydroxide solution neutralizes acids forming the corresponding calcium salts.

$$Ca(OH)_2 + 2HCl \longrightarrow CaCl_2 + 2H_2O$$

Calcium hydroxide solution (lime water) absorbs carbon dioxide and forms calcium carbonate.

$$Ca(OH)_2 + CO_2 + H_2O \longrightarrow CaCO_3 + 2H_2O$$

This is the reaction in which lime water is turned milky by the passing of carbon dioxide. This is a test for carbonates and bicarbonates.

When calcium hydroxide is strongly heated, calcium oxide is formed.

$$Ca(OH)_2 \xrightarrow{\Delta} CaO + H_2O$$

It is official in I.P.

Official Tests for Identity

A solution of the sample in acetic acid gives the reactions of calcium (see Chapter 13).

Standard: It contains not less than 90% of Ca (OH)$_2$.

Storage Condition: Since it absorbs carbon dioxide from the atmosphere and is converted into calcium carbonate, it must be stored in tightly closed containers.

Chemical Incompatibility: Since it is a weak base, it will react with acids. However this is turned into an advantage in the preparation of zinc cream. In this the calcium hydroxide solution is reacted with oleic acid to form calcium oleate which, being a divalent soap, produces a water in oil emulsion of the arachis oil and water.

Medicinal and Pharmaceutical Uses

Astringent: It may be used as an antacid also. Because of its alkalinity and consequent soap forming property, it may be used as in zinc cream above. Lime water (which is a saturated solution of calcium hydroxide in water) is used as a reagent in the laboratory for testing for the presence of carbon dioxide which turns lime water milky. Calcium hydroxide solution is also used in the assay of opium. Soda lime (fused granules of sodium hydroxide and calcium hydroxide) is used in closed circuit anaesthetic apparatus to absorb exhaled carbon dioxide.

CHAPTER 3
ANTIOXIDANTS

Antioxidants can also be called as preservatives in the sense that they preserve a product from being oxidised and consequently spoiled. Substances which are easily oxidised are unsaturated compounds, phenols, vitamins etc. and they require the addition of antioxidants to guard against oxidation. Antioxidants are usually reducing agents and they get oxidised more readily by combining with the oxygen or oxidizing agent themselves. Thus they preserve the medicament to which they are added. Nitrogen being inert chemically replaces oxygen in containers of drugs and thus preserves drugs from oxidation.

1. HYPOPHOSPHOROUS ACID, H_3PO_2

Preparation: It is prepared by decomposing a boiled aqueous solution of calcium hypophosphite with oxalic acid.

$$Ca(PH_2O_2)_2 + H_2C_2O_4 \longrightarrow CaC_2O_4 + 2HPH_2O_3 \text{ or } 2\,H_3PO_2$$

Calcium   Oxalic acid   Cal.oxalate   Hypophosphorus acid.
hypophosphite

The insoluble calcium oxalate is filtered off and the filtrate containing the hypophosphorous acid is concentrated in vacuum to give white crystals of the acid.

Physical and Chemical Properties

Pure hypophosphorous acid is a colourless, crystalline solid. It is readily soluble in water. Usually it is available as a colourless or slightly yellow liquid without odour containing about 31% of H_3PO_2.

It is a strong monobasic acid. Only one of three hydrogen atoms in its structure is ionizable.

$$H_3PO_2 \rightleftharpoons H^+ + H_2PO_2^-.$$

It forms salts known as hypophosphites by reacting with metals or metallic hydroxides or carbonates.

$$Zn + 2H_3PO_2 \longrightarrow Zn(H_2PO_2)_2 + H_2\uparrow$$
$$H_3PO_2 + Na_2CO_3 \longrightarrow 2NaH_2PO_2 + H_2O + CO_2\uparrow$$

It is a powerful reducing agent.

When it is treated with copper sulphate solution and heated to $60^\circ C$, a reddish precipitate of cuprous hydride is formed.

$$2CuSO_4 + 2H_3PO_2 + 4H_2O \longrightarrow 2H_3PO_4 + Cu_2H_2\downarrow$$
$$\text{Cuprous hydride}$$
$$+ 2H_2SO_4 + H_2\uparrow$$

When the solution is boiled, the cuprous hydride decomposes to metallic copper and hydrogen.

When it is mixed with acidified potassium permanganate solution, it reduces the permanganate and the pink colour is discharged.

$$5H_3PO_2 + 4KMnO_4 + 6H_2SO_4 \longrightarrow 2K_2SO_4 + 4MnSO_4$$
$$+ 5H_3PO_4 + 6H_2O.$$

Mercuric chloride mixed with hypophosphorus acid is reduced first to white mercurous chloride and finally to mercury.

On strong heating, it decomposes to phosphorous acid and phosphine.

$$3H_3PO_2 \xrightarrow{\Delta} PH_3\uparrow + 2H_3PO_3.$$
$$\text{Phosphine} \quad \text{Phosphorous acid.}$$

Storage Condition: Since it is a powerful reducing agent, it will react with oxygen of the atmosphere and get oxidised. So it must be kept in tightly closed containers.

Chemical Incompatibility: As a strong acid, it will react with all bases and alkalis. Secondly it is a reducing agent and will reduce any substance prone to reduction and also all oxidizing agents.

Medicinal or Pharmaceutical Use: Its use in pharmacy is only as a reducing agent. Thus it is used in Syrup of Ferrous Iodide preparation. Here all the ferric iodide present is reduced to ferrous iodide by the hypophosphorous acid so that the preparation contains only ferrous iodide.

2. SULPHUR DIOXIDE, SO_2

Preparation

1. Sulphur dioxide is produced when sulphur is burnt in air or oxygen.

$$S + O_2 \xrightarrow{\Delta} SO_2\uparrow$$

A small quantity of sulphur trioxide also is produced.

2. Sulphur dioxide is also produced by roasting metallic sulphides in air.

$$4FeS_2 + 11O_2 \xrightarrow{\Delta} 2Fe_2O_3 + 8SO_2\uparrow$$

$$Cu_2S + 2O_2 \xrightarrow{\Delta} 2CuO + SO_2\uparrow$$

3. It is also produced by reducing sulphuric acid with carbon or sulphur or copper.

$$2H_2SO_4 + Cu \longrightarrow SO_2\uparrow + CuSO_4 + 2H_2O.$$

Physical and Chemical Properties

Sulphur dioxide is a colourless gas with a pungent and irritating odour. It is non-inflammable and is soluble in water. Its aqueous solution is acid to litmus since sulphurous acid is formed. It is stable even at high temperatures.

However under the influence of a catalyst, it combines with oxygen to form sulphur trioxide.

$$SO_2 + O \longrightarrow SO_3$$

In direct sunlight as well as in the presence of a catalyst like camphor, sulphur dioxide forms addition compounds. It also forms a hydrate with 7 molecules of water ($SO_2.7H_2O$). The hydrate is obtained by cooling a saturated aqueous solution of sulphur dioxide.

It is a good reducing agent. It reduces iodine and chlorine. It reduces potassium iodate to iodine and also discharges the colour of potassium permanganate solution.

$$I_2 + 2H_2O + SO_2 \longrightarrow H_2SO_4 + 2HI$$

$$SO_2 + Cl_2 \longrightarrow SO_2Cl_2$$
$$\text{Sulphuryl chloride}$$
$$2KIO_3 + 4H_2O + 5SO_2 \longrightarrow 2KHSO_4 + I_2 + 3H_2SO_4$$
$$2KMnO_4 + 2H_2O + 5SO_2 \longrightarrow K_2SO_4 + 2MnSO_4 + 2H_2SO_4$$

Tests for Identity

1. Sulphur dioxide has a characteristic, acrid odour.

2. Filter paper moistened with potassium iodate and starch solutions and dried and exposed to sulphur dioxide develops a blue colour. On continuous exposure, the blue colour disappears.

    This is due to the fact that potassium iodate is reduced to iodine by sulphur dioxide and the iodine gives the blue colour with starch. However on further exposure, the sulphur dioxide reduces iodine to hydrogen iodide (HI) and the blue colour disappears.

3. When moistened mercuric nitrate paper is brought into contact with sulphur dioxide, it turns black due to the reduction of mercuric nitrate to mercury.

Storage Condition: Since sulphur dioxide is a powerful reducing agent, it reacts with oxygen of the atmosphere. Further it is also a gas. So it should be stored in a tightly closed container, preferably a cylinder.

Medicinal and Pharmaceutical Uses: Formerly sulphur dioxide was used as an antioxidant preservative because of its reducing action in certain easily oxidisable preparations. However it finds extensive use in bleaching wood pulp and straw. It is also used for fumigating rooms and in the manufacture of sugar and sulphuric acid.

3. SODIUM BISULPHITE, $NaHSO_3$

Preparation: Sodium bisulphite is prepared by passing sulphur dioxide into a solution of sodium carbonate till the solution is saturated with sulphur dioxide. First the sulphur dioxide dissolves in water to form sulphurous acid which reacts with sodium carbonate to give sodium bisulphite.

$$SO_2 + H_2O \longrightarrow H_2SO_3$$

$$Na_2CO_3 + 2H_2SO_3 \longrightarrow 2NaHSO_3 + H_2O + CO_2\uparrow$$

Sodium bisulphite may be crystallized from the solution directly. Alternatively it may be precipitated as a white powder by the addition of alcohol.

Physical and Chemical Properties

Sodium bisulphite is a white powder or it may occur as white crystals. It has the odour of sulphur dioxide. It is soluble in water.

It reacts with acids to yield sulphurous acid.

$$NaHSO_3 + HCl \longrightarrow NaCl + H_2SO_3$$

It is a powerful reducing agent and reduces in acid solution iodine, permanganate, dichromate, halogens, hydrogen peroxide, ferric salts etc. itself getting oxidised to sodium bisulphate. The reaction with iodine is given below.

$$NaHSO_3 + I_2 + H_2O \longrightarrow NaHSO_4 + 2HI$$

Actually this is the assay method for sodium bisulphite.

Sodium bisulphite is sufficiently acidic to produce effervescence with sodium carbonate. Sodium sulphite is formed.

$$2NaHSO_3 + Na_2CO_3 \longrightarrow 2Na_2SO_3 + H_2O + CO_2\uparrow$$

Sodium bisulphite forms addition compounds with organic compounds containing carbonyl groups such as aldehydes and ketones.

$$\diagdown C = O + NaHSO_3 \rightarrow \diagdown C \diagup\!\!\!\diagdown^{OH}_{SO_3Na}$$

The organic compound is now converted into a water-soluble, stable form which can be dissolved in water and injected.

Tests for Identity

1. Sodium bisulphite solution in water gives the reactions of sodium (see Chapter 13).

2. A solution of sodium bisulphite treated with hydrochloric acid turns a filter paper moistened with mercurous nitrate solution black.

Sodium bisulphite liberates sulphur dioxide on treatment with hydrochloric acid and the sulphur dioxide reduces mercurous nitrate to mercury.

Storage Condition: Sodium bisulphite is somewhat unstable in air releasing sulphur dioxide. So it should be stored in a tightly closed container.

Chemical Incompatibility: Since sodium bisulphite is a powerful reducing agent, it is incompatible with all substances liable to be reduced and also with all oxidizing agents such as permanganate, dichromate, iodine, hydrogen peroxide, halogens, hypochlorous acid, ferric salts etc.

Medicinal and Pharmaceutical Uses: Formerly sodium bisulphite was used as an antioxidant preservative in a concentration of 0.1-0.2% in certain injections such as adrenalin injection and phenylephrine injection. Now sodium metabisulphite has replaced sodium bisulphite in these preparations. As already stated sodium bisulphite is used to convert certain ketonic compounds into soluble sodium bisulphite compounds.

4. SODIUM METABISULPHITE, $Na_2S_2O_5$

Preparation: Sodium metabisulphite is produced by passing sulphur dioxide into a hot concentrated sodium hydroxide solution and saturating it. Sodium bisulphite which is first formed is converted into sodium metabisulphite.

$$NaOH + SO_2 \longrightarrow NaHSO_3$$
$$2NaHSO_3 \rightleftharpoons Na_2S_2O_5 + H_2O$$

Physical and Chemical Properties: Sodium metabisulphite occurs as colourless, prismatic crystals or as a white powder which may become yellowish on keeping. It has a sulphurous odour and an acid and saline taste. It contains one molecule of water of hydration. It effloresces and slowly gets oxidized to sulphate on exposure to air. It is acid in reaction and is also a powerful reducing agent. It is freely soluble in water.

On heating it decomposes into sodium sulphite and sulphur dioxide and for this reason may be considered as sodium sulphite with excess of sulphur dioxide to explain its reducing action.

$$Na_2S_2O_5 \longrightarrow Na_2SO_3 + SO_2\uparrow$$

It reduces iodine, permanganate, dichromate, ferric salts etc. Its reaction with iodine is used as the assay method.

$$2I_2 + Na_2S_2O_5 + 3H_2O \longrightarrow 4HI + 2NaHSO_4$$

It is official in I.P.

Official Tests for Identity

1. Yields the reactions characteristic of sodium salts.

2. A solution of the sample decolourises iodine solution and the resulting solution gives the reactions of sulphates.

Standard: Contains not less than 95% of $Na_2S_2O_5$.

Storage Condition: Sodium metabisulphite should be kept in a tightly closed container. On exposure to air and moisture it is slowly oxidised to sulphate with disintegration of crystals. It is also efflorescent.

Chemical Incompatibility: Since it is acidic, it is incompatible with bases. Since it is also a good reducing agent, it is incompatible with oxidizing agents.

Medicinal and Pharmaceutical Use

Antioxidant Preservative: It is used to stabilize injections of adrenalin tartrate and morphine and also adrenaline solution. It is also used in the preparation of photographic developers and as an antichlor after bleaching paper or cloth with chlorine.

5. SODIUM THIOSULPHATE, $Na_2S_2O_3.5H_2O$

Preparation: 1. One half of a concentrated solution of sodium carbonate is saturated with sulphur dioxide and the other half is added to it. Sodium sulphite is formed.

$$Na_2CO_3 + 2SO_2 + H_2O \longrightarrow 2NaHSO_3 + CO_2\uparrow$$
$$2NaHSO_3 + Na_2CO_3 \longrightarrow Na_2SO_3 + H_2O + CO_2\uparrow$$

Sodium thiosulphate solution is prepared by boiling sodium sulphite solution with flowers of sulphur and stirring till the alkaline reaction has disappeared.

$$Na_2SO_3 + S \longrightarrow Na_2S_2O_3$$

The excess of sulphur is filtered off and the filtrate evaporated to crystallization when crystals of sodium thiosulphate ($Na_2S_2O_3.5H_2O$) separate on slow cooling.

2. It can also be prepared by passing sulphur dioxide into sodium sulphide solution.

$$2Na_2S + 3SO_2 \longrightarrow 2Na_2S_2O_3 + S$$

Physical and Chemical Properties

Sodium thiosulphate occurs as large, colourless, monoclinic crystals or as a coarse, crystalline powder. It is odourless and has a saline taste. It is deliquescent in moist air and effloresces in dry air at temperatures above $33^{\circ}C$. It is very soluble in water and insoluble in alcohol. Aqueous neutral or alkaline solutions of the salt decompose on boiling because of reduction to sulphide and oxidation to sulphate.

At $56^{\circ}C$ the salt melts in its water of hydration and at $100^{\circ}C$ it become anhydrous. At $100^{\circ}C$ decomposition of the salt begins and at $220^{\circ}C$ it is completely converted into sulphur, sulphur dioxide, sodium sulphide and sodium sulphate.

$$4\,Na_2S_2O_3 \xrightarrow{\Delta} 3Na_2SO_4 + Na_2S_5.$$

$$Na_2S_5 \xrightarrow{\Delta} Na_2S + 4S$$

$$Na_2S_5 + 4O_2 \xrightarrow{\Delta} Na_2S + 4SO_2.$$

Addition of a mineral acid such as hydrochloric acid to a solution of sodium thiosulphate produces thiosulphuric acid which immediately decomposes into sulphur, sulphur dioxide and water.

$$Na_2S_2O_3 + 2HCl \longrightarrow H_2S_2O_3\downarrow + 2NaCl$$
$$\text{Thiosulphuric acid}$$

$$H_2S_2O_3 \longrightarrow S\downarrow + SO_2\uparrow + H_2O$$

Silver nitrate gives with a very dilute solution of sodium thiosulphate a white precipitate which quickly changes colour to yellow, brown and finally black due to the formation of silver sulphide.

$$Na_2S_2O_3 + 2AgNO_3 \longrightarrow Ag_2S_2O_3 \downarrow + 2NaNO_3$$
Silver thiosulphate
(white)

$$Ag_2S_2O_3 + H_2O \longrightarrow Ag_2S + H_2SO_4$$
Silver sulphide
(black)

Sodium thiosulphate is a good reducing agent and reduces halogens such as chlorine and iodine. It decolourises iodine solution and this is the method by which both iodine and sodium thiosulphate are assayed.

$$2Na_2S_2O_3 + I_2 \longrightarrow 2NaI + Na_2S_4O_6$$
Sodium tetrathionate.

Upon the addition of a few drops of ferric chloride solution to a solution of sodium thiosulphate, a red colour appears and the colour disappears quickly. The red colour is due to the formation of ferric thiosulphate and the disappearance of the colour is due to the reduction of the ferric salt by the sodium thiosulphate.

A moderately concentrated solution of sodium thiosulphate gives a white precipitate of barium thiosulphate with barium chloride. No precipitate is obtained with calcium chloride since calcium thiosulphate is fairly soluble in water.

$$Na_2S_2O_3 + BaCl_2 \longrightarrow BaS_2O_3 + 2NaCl$$

It is official in I.P.

Official Tests for Identity

1. To a solution in water are added a few drops of iodine solution. The colour is discharged.

2. A solution in water gives the reactions of sodium and of thiosulphates (see Chapter 13).

Non-official Tests for Identity

1. To a solution in water, dilute hydrochloric acid is added. A white precipitate of sulphur which soon changes to yellow is obtained. Sulphur dioxide is liberated.

2. Addition of Ferric Chloride, T.S.to a solution in water gives a dark violet colour which quickly disappears.

Standard: Sodium thiosulphate contains not less than 99 per cent and not more than the equivalent of 101 percent of $Na_2S_2O_3 .5H_2O$.

Storage Condition: Since it is deliquescent in moist air and efflorescent in dry air, it must be stored in tightly closed, air tight containers.

Chemical Incompatibility: Sodium thiosulphate is incompatible with acids, silver nitrate, halogens such as chlorine and iodine, ferric salts and barium chloride.

Assay: A solution in water is titrated with N/10 iodine solution using starch solution as indicator. Appearance of a permanent blue colour is the end point.

Medicinal and Pharmaceutical Uses

Antidote to Cyanide Poisoning: It is also used as an antifungal agent. Sometimes it is used as a cathartic. Due to its property of dissolving silver halides, it is used in photography for fixing under the name 'hypo'. During bleaching of textiles, it is used as an antichlor (that is, to remove excess of chlorine). It is also used in the extraction of gold and silver from their ores.

6. SODIUM NITRITE, NaNO₂

Preparation: Sodium nitrite is usually obtained by reducing sodium nitrate.

1. By reducing sodium nitrate with carbon in the presence of lime which removes carbon dioxide as calcium carbonate.

$$2NaNO_3 + C + Ca(OH)_2 \longrightarrow 2NaNO_2 + CaCO_3 + H_2O.$$

2. By reducing sodium nitrate with lead at 450 to $500^{\circ}C$ or better still with sulphur and sodium hydroxide.

$$NaNO_3 + Pb \longrightarrow NaNO_2 + PbO$$

$$3NaNO_3 + 2NaOH + S \longrightarrow 3NaNO_2 + Na_2SO_4 + H_2O.$$

Physical and Chemical Properties

Sodium nitrite occurs as colourless to slightly yellow crystals or as a slightly yellow, granular powder. It is odourless and has a mild, saline taste. When exposed to the atmosphere, it deliquesces and is slowly oxidised to sodium nitrate. It is freely soluble in water and sparingly soluble in alcohol.

Aqueous solutions of sodium nitrite are alkaline because it is the salt of a weak acid (nitrous acid) and is appreciably hydrolyzed in solution. Sodium nitrite is easily decomposed by acidification with dilute sulphuric acid to give nitric oxide (NO) which is readily oxidised by atmospheric oxygen to form nitrogen peroxide (NO_2).

$$2NaNO_2 + H_2SO_4 \longrightarrow Na_2SO_4 + 2HNO_2$$
$$3HNO_3 \longrightarrow H_2O + 2NO + HNO_3$$
$$2NO + O_2 \longrightarrow 2NO_2\uparrow$$

It behaves both as an oxidizing agent and as a reducing agent.

a. **As an oxidizing Agent**: It oxidizes acidified potassium iodide to iodine and bleaches indigo. It oxidizes also stannous chloride to stannic chloride.

$$2HNO_2 + 2KI + H_2SO_4 \longrightarrow I_2 + 2NO\uparrow + 2H_2O + K_2SO_4.$$

b. **As a reducing Agent**: It reduces acidified potassium permanganate and potassium dichromate solutions.

$$5NaNO_2 + 2KMnO_4 + 3H_2SO_4 \longrightarrow 5NaNO_3 + K_2SO_4 + 2MnSO_4 + 3H_2O.$$

In this reaction the sodium nitrite is oxidised to sodium nitrate. This is the assay method for sodium nitrite. The known excess of pot.permanganate solution added is back titrated with decinormal oxalic acid solution.

It is official in I.P.1966.

Tests for Identity

1. A solution in water gives the reactions of sodium and of nitrites.(See Chapter 13).

2. When sodium nitrite is treated with mineral acids or acetic acid, it gives brownish red fumes of nitrogen dioxide.

3. A solution of sodium nitrite in water, when added to potassium iodide containing a little starch solution, gives a blue colour. This is due to the oxidation of potassium iodide to iodine which gives the blue colour with starch.

Storage Condition: Since sodium nitrite is deliquescent and is slowly oxidised to sodium nitrate on exposure to atmosphere, it should be stored in tightly closed containers.

Chemical Incompatibility: Sodium nitrite is incompatible with acids, certain oxidizing agents and also with potassium iodide. It is also incompatible with some reducing agents.

Medicinal and Pharmaceutical Uses

Antidote to Cyanide Poisoning: Sodium nitrite combines with haemoglobin of the blood to form methaemoglobin with which the cyanide forms cyanmethaemoglobin. In this form the cyanide is not toxic to the body. After the administration of nitrite, sodium thiosulphate is injected to convert the cyanide further to thiocyanate which is also not toxic.

Sodium nitrite is used as a vasodilator but rarely nowadays in view of its slow onset of action. It is also used in the manufacture of azo dyes and as a reagent in the laboratory.

7. NITROGEN, N_2

Nitrogen occurs in the atmosphere to the extent of 70 per cent. It also occurs in large quantities as white salt petre ($NaNO_3$). Combined with hydrogen it occurs as ammonia and also in organic combination as proteins, aminoacids, alkaloids etc. in plant and animal tissues. It is also present as nitrates in the soil formed by the soil bacteria such as the nitrifying bacteria.

Preparation: Nitrogen may be obtained either by removing the oxygen from the atmospheric air or by decomposing compounds in which it may occur:

(a). Burning phosphorus in air in a closed container.

(b). Passing air over red-hot copper filings.

(c). Passing air through a solution of sodium hydrosulphite ($Na_2S_2O_4$) which will absorb oxygen, and (d). Shaking an alkaline solution of pyrogallol with air. Alkaline solution of pyrogallol absorbs oxygen.

Nitrogen may also be prepared by fractional distillation of liquid air.

Chemically nitrogen is also prepared by oxidation of ammonia with red hot copper oxide.

$$2NH_3 + 3CuO \longrightarrow N_2 + 3H_2O + 3Cu$$

Physical and Chemical Properties

Nitrogen is a colourless, odourless and tasteless gas. It is slightly lighter than air. It is only slightly soluble in water. It is not poisonous but animals die in an atmosphere of nitrogen for lack of oxygen. It can be liquefied to a colourless liquid boiling at $-195.8°C$. Nitrogen neither burns itself nor supports combustion.

Nitrogen is a very inert gas. It combines with other elements only with difficulty. With oxygen it combines only in the presence of lightning or when the mixture is passed through an electric arc.

$$N_2 + O_2 \rightleftharpoons 2NO$$

With hydrogen it combines under a pressure of 200–900 atmospheres and in the presence of a catalyst made of finely divided iron and molybdenum at $452°C$.

$$N_2 + 3H_2 \rightleftharpoons 2NH_3$$

Even though nitrogen is non-combustible and is also not a supporter of combustion, burning magnesium or aluminium continues to burn in an atmosphere of nitrogen forming the corresponding nitride.

$$3Mg + N_2 \longrightarrow Mg_2N_2$$
$$\text{Magnesium nitride}$$

If the ash containing the nitride is moistened with water, the nitride is hydrolysed and the ammonia formed can be tested with red litmus.

$$Mg_2N_2 + 6H_2O \longrightarrow 3Mg(OH)_2 + 2NH_3\uparrow$$

Tests for Identity

1. Nitrogen is colourless, odourless and tasteless.
2. Nitrogen has no action on litmus and lime water.
3. The flame of a burning wood splinter when introduced into nitrogen is extinguished (put out).
4. Burning magnesium ribbon continues to burn in a jar of nitrogen.

Storage Condition: Since nitrogen is a gas, it must be stored under pressure in a gas cylinder tightly closed.

Chemical Incompatibility: Since nitrogen is very inert, it does not react with other elements or compounds readily.

Medicinal and Pharmaceutical Uses: Its usual pharmaceutical use is to retard or prevent oxidation by providing an inert atmosphere in the containers containing certain medicaments such as ergometrine injection, some vitamin preparations and some fish liver oils. In these containers, the air is replaced by nitrogen.

It is also used for filling electric lamps. It is used in the manufacture of ammonia, nitric acid, calcium cyanamide and other nitrogen compounds. Liquid nitrogen is used to freeze water etc. Mercury thermometers used above $200^{o}C$ have nitrogen filled above the mercury column to decrease the evaporation of mercury and also to prevent its oxidation.

CHAPTER 4

GASTROINTESTINAL AGENTS

Gastrointestinal agents are drugs which produce different effects in the gastrointestinal tract.

A. ACIDIFYING AGENT

DILUTE HYDROCHLORIC ACID, HCl

Preparation: Dilute Hydrochloric Acid is prepared from Hydrochloric Acid, I.P./B.P.by diluting 274 g of the acid with 726 g of purified water.

Physical and Chemical Properties

Dilute hydrochloric acid is a clear, colourless liquid with an acid taste. Its chemical properties are the same as those given under Hydrochloric Acid (refer Chapter 2). It is official in the I.P.

Official Tests for Identity

1. Gives the reactions characteristic of chlorides (refer Chapter 13).

2. The solution is strongly acidic (test with any indicator).

Standard: Dilute Hydrochloric Acid contains not less than 9.5 percent w/w and not more than 10.5 percent w/w of HCl.

Storage Condition: It should be kept in a stoppered container of glass or other inert material and stored at a temperature not exceeding 30oC.

Chemical Incompatibility and Assay

Refer Hydrochloric Acid (Chapter 2).

Medicinal and Pharmaceutical Uses

Acidifier. Dilute hydrochloric acid is administered orally to treat achlorhydria (lack of hydrochloric acid in the gastric juice). The dose is 0.6 to 8 ml(I.P.) It is also used as a reagent in the laboratory.

35

B. ANTACIDS

Antacids are drugs used to neutralize the hydrochloric acid secreted in the stomach in the gastric juice.

1. SODIUM BICARBONATE, NaHCO₃

Preparation: Sodium bicarbonate may be made by the ammonia soda process for sodium carbonate. However this does not give medicinal grade sodium bicarbonate. Therefore to obtain medicinal grade sodium bicarbonate the sample is heated to get sodium carbonate. Then sodium carbonate is dissolved in water and carbon dioxide is passed through it. Sodium bicarbonate is precipitated and it is washed and dried.

$$Na_2CO_3 + CO_2 + H_2O \longrightarrow 2NaHCO_3.$$

(a) **Physical Properties:** Sodium bicarbonate is a white, odourless, crystalline, monoclinic powder. It is stable in dry air, but in moist air it slowly decomposes to sodium carbonate, carbon dioxide and water. It is soluble 1 in 10 in water. It is insoluble in alcohol.

(b) **Chemical Properties:**

1. When heated dry or in solution in water, it loses water and carbon dioxide and forms the normal carbonate.

$$2NaHCO_3 \longrightarrow Na_2CO_3 + H_2O + CO_2$$

2. Carbon dioxide is again liberated when it is treated with any acid:

$$NaHCO_3 + HCl \longrightarrow NaCl + CO_2 + H_2O.$$

3. Aqueous solutions of sodium bicarbonate are slightly alkaline, as the bicarbonate ion is hydrolyzed in solution.

$$HCO_{3-} + H_2O \longrightarrow H_2CO_3 + OH^-$$

However it is so slightly alkaline that it fails to turn phenolphthalein red. This distinguishes sodium bicarbonate from sodium carbonate. It is official in I.P.

Official Tests for Identity

Gives the reactions characteristic of sodium and bicarbonates (see Chapter 13).

Standard: Contains between 99 and 100.5 percent of $NaHCO_3$.

Storage Condition: Since it slowly decomposes in moist air, store in a well-closed container in a cool place.

Chemical Incompatibility

Since sodium bicarbonate is a base, it is incompatible with acids which release carbon dioxide from it. Carbon dioxide may also be evolved when sodium bicarbonate is mixed with borax and glycerin or bismuth subnitrate or calcium and magnesium salts. Sodium bicarbonate may also liberate some alkaloids from their salt solutions.

Assay: An accurately weighed quantity is dissolved in water and titrated with N/2 sulphuric acid using methyl orange as indicator.

$$H_2SO_4 + 2NaHCO_3 \longrightarrow Na_2SO_4 + 2H_2O + 2CO_2\uparrow$$

Medicinal and Pharmaceutical Uses

Sodium bicarbonate may be used as an **antacid**. Since it quickly neutralizes the gastric acid, the stomach secretes more acid to maintain the acid pH. This is what is known as "rebound acidity" and this may even lead to peptic ulcer. However, sodium bicarbonate can be used as a good antacid, if used in controlled doses.

Sodium bicarbonate may also be given by injection to relieve acidosis in the blood, especially in diabetic coma. So it is a **systemic alkaliser**. It is also an **electrolyte replenisher**.

2. CALCIUM CARBONATE, $CaCO_3$

Preparation: Calcium carbonate is prepared by passing carbon dioxide through lime water (calcium hydroxide solution).

$$Ca(OH)_2 + CO_2 \longrightarrow CaCO_3\downarrow + H_2O$$

However calcium carbonate is usually prepared by mixing boiling sodium carbonate and calcium chloride solutions and the resulting precipitate is allowed to subside.

$$CaCl_2 + Na_2CO_3 \longrightarrow CaCO_3\downarrow + 2NaCl.$$

The precipitated calcium carbonate is collected on a calico filter, washed with boiling water till it is free from chloride and dried.

Physical and Chemical Properties

Calcium carbonate is a fine, white, microcrystalline powder which is odourless and tasteless. It is practically insoluble in water but slightly soluble in water containing carbon dioxide or any ammonium salt. This is because it forms the bicarbonate with carbon dioxide and the bicarbonate is slightly soluble in water. Excepting ammonium carbonate and bicarbonate, all the other ammonium salts are acidic and give effervescence with calcium carbonate.

$$CaCO_3 + CO_2 + H_2O \longrightarrow Ca(HCO_3)_2$$
$$\text{Calcium bicarbonate}$$

$$CaCO_3 + 2NH_4Cl \longrightarrow CaCl_2 + 2NH_3 + H_2O + CO_2\uparrow$$

It is insoluble in alcohol but soluble in most acids with effervescence.

$$CaCO_3 + 2HCl \longrightarrow CaCl_2 + CO_2\uparrow + H_2O$$

It is stable in air. It is official in I.P.

Calcium carbonate is the most abundant calcium salt occurring in nature. It occurs as chalk, limestone, marble, calcite and aragonite. It is amorphous in chalk whereas it is in irregular crystals in limestone. It is crystalline in marble, calcite and aragonite. Calcite occurs as hexagonal crystals and aragonite as rhombic crystals.

Official Tests for Identity: A solution of the substance in acetic acid, which is boiled, gives the reactions of calcium (see Chapter 13).

Standard: Calcium carbonate is precipitated calcium carbonate. It is also known as precipitated chalk. It contains not less than 98 per cent of $CaCO_3$, calculated with reference to the dried substance.

Storage Condition: Since it is stable in air, it may be stored in a well closed container.

Chemical Incompatibility: Calcium carbonate is incompatible with acids and ammonium salts except ammonium carbonate and ammonium bicarbonate. It is also incompatible with borax and glycerin. In all these reactions carbon dioxide is evolved.

Medicinal and Pharmaceutical Uses

Antacid: Precipitated chalk is used as a dentifrice (tooth powder).

Prepared chalk (made by the process of elutriation) is usually used in preference to precipitated chalk as an antacid. Because of its mild, non-irritating nature, it is also used in the treatment of some forms of diarrhoea.

Limestone is used in the manufacture of cement, lime, washing soda and glass.

3. MAGNESIUM CARBONATE

Magnesium carbonate occurs in two forms, that is, heavy magnesium carbonate and light magnesium carbonate. They are both hydrated basic magnesium carbonates and differ only in the content of water of hydration (the heavy variety having $4H_2O$ and the light one with $3H_2O$) and in the bulk density.

HEAVY MAGNESIUM CARBONATE, $3MgCO_3, Mg(OH)_2, 4H_2O$

Preparation: Crystalline magnesium sulphate (125 parts) and crystalline sodium carbonate (150 parts) each dissolved in 250 parts of boiling water are mixed together and evaporated to dryness. The residue is digested with boiling water for half an hour. The precipitate of heavy magnesium carbonate is collected on a calico filter, washed till sulphate is fully removed and dried in a water-oven.

$$4MgSO_4 . 7H_2O + 4Na_2CO_3. 10H_2O \rightarrow 3MgCO_3. Mg(OH)_2. 4H_2O$$
$$+ 4Na_2SO_4 + CO_2\uparrow + 63H_2O$$

Physical and Chemical Properties

Heavy magnesium carbonate is a white, granular powder without odour and taste. It is practically insoluble in water and in alcohol. It is soluble in dilute acids with effervescence. 15 g of heavy magnesium carbonate occupy a volume of about 30 ml. It is stable in air.

Because of its insolubility in most solvents, it is quite inert chemically. When heavy magnesium carbonate is treated with dilute hydrochloric acid, carbon dioxide is evolved.

$$3MgCO_3. Mg(OH)_2. 4H_2O + 8HCl \longrightarrow 4MgCl_2 + 3CO_2\uparrow$$
$$+ 9H_2O.$$

When heated to redness, it loses carbon dioxide and water and leaves a residue of heavy magnesium oxide.

$$3 \, MgCO_3. \, Mg(OH)_2. \, 4H_2O \xrightarrow{\Delta} 4MgO + 3CO_2\uparrow + 5H_2O.$$

By heating in solution with sodium bicarbonate, the normal carbonate ($MgCO_3$) is formed. It is official in I.P.

Official Tests for Identity

A solution in dilute nitric acid gives the reactions of magnesium and of carbonates (see Chapter 13).

Non-official Test for Identity

When magnesium carbonate is treated with dilute hydrochloric acid, carbon dioxide is evolved.

Standard: It contains the equivalent of not less than 40 per cent and not more than 45 per cent of MgO.

Storage Condition: Since it is stable in air, store in a well closed container.

Chemical Incompatibility: It is incompatible with acids and with soluble bicarbonates.

Medicinal and Pharmaceutical Uses

Antacid and Laxative: It is used as a clarifying or filtering agent for alkaline solutions (e.g.:Tolu Syrup). It is also used as an abrasive in some tooth powders.

LIGHT MAGNESIUM CARBONATE, $3MgCO_3$, $Mg(OH)_2.3H_2O$

Preparation: Crystalline magnesium sulphate (125 parts) and crystalline sodium carbonate (150 parts) are dissolved separately in 1000 ml cold water each and mixed. Then the solution is boiled for fifteen minutes. The precipitate of light magnesium carbonate is collected on a calico filter, washed free from sulphate and dried in a water-oven.

$$4MgSO_4 . 7H_2O + 4Na_2CO_3. \, 10H_2O \rightarrow 3MgCO_3. \, Mg(OH)_2. \, 3H_2O$$
$$+ \, 4Na_2SO_4 + CO_2\uparrow + 64H_2O$$

Physical and Chemical Properties

Light magnesium carbonate is a very light, white powder which is without odour. It is almost tasteless. It is practically insoluble in water and in alcohol. It is soluble in dilute acids with effervescence. 15 g of light magnesium carbonate occupy a volume of about 125 ml.

When heated to redness, it loses carbon dioxide and water and leaves a residue of light magnesium oxide.

$$3MgCO_3.Mg(OH)_2 3H_2O \xrightarrow{\Delta} 4MgO + 3CO_2\uparrow + 4H_2O.$$

Other chemical properties are the same as for heavy magnesium carbonate. It is official in I.P.

Official Tests for Identity	}	
Non-official Test for Identity	}	Same as for
Standard	}	Heavy Magnesium
Storage Condition	}	Carbonate
Medicinal and Pharmaceutical Uses	}	

4. MAGNESIUM OXIDE, MgO

Magnesium oxide occurs in two forms, that is, heavy magnesium oxide and light magnesium oxide. They differ in bulk density only and the bulk of a definite weight of light magnesium oxide is about three and a half times more than that of the same weight of heavy magnesium oxide.

HEAVY MAGNESIUM OXIDE, MgO

Preparation: Heavy magnesium oxide is prepared by heating the heavy magnesium carbonate to dull redness till carbon dioxide is no longer evolved.

$$3MgCO_3Mg(OH)_2.4H_2O \xrightarrow{\Delta} 4MgO + 3CO_2\uparrow + 5H_2O$$

The residue is heavy magnesium oxide.

Physical and Chemical Properties

It is a dense, white powder which is odourless and slightly alkaline. It is practically insoluble in water and in alcohol. It is soluble

41

in dilute acids. 15 g of heavy magnesium oxide occupy a volume of about 30 ml.

Upon exposure to air, it absorbs carbon dioxide and moisture and is converted to the basic carbonates. It is official in I.P.

Official Tests for Identity

A solution in nitric acid gives the reactions of magnesium (see Chapter 13).

Standard: Heavy Magnesium Oxide contains not less than 98 per cent of MgO, calculated with reference to the substance ignited at 900°C.

Storage condition: Since it absorbs carbon dioxide and moisture from the air, store in tightly closed containers.

Chemical Incompatibility: It is incompatible with acids.

Medicinal and Pharmaceutical Uses. Antacid and Laxative.

LIGHT MAGNESIUM OXIDE, MgO

Preparation: Light magnesium oxide is prepared by heating the light magnesium carbonate to dull redness till carbon dioxide is no longer evolved.

$$3MgCO_3.Mg(OH)_2.3H_2O \xrightarrow{\Delta} 4MgO + 3CO_2\uparrow + 4H_2O.$$

The residue is light magnesium oxide.

Physical and Chemical Properties

Light magnesium Oxide is a very light, white powder which is odourless and slightly alkaline. It is soluble in dilute acids. 15 g of light magnesium oxide occupy a volume of about 150 ml. It is practically insoluble in water but soluble in alcohol. Upon exposure to air, it also absorbs carbon dioxide and moisture and is converted to the basic carbonates. It is official in I.P.

Official Tests for Identity	}
Standard	} Same as for Heavy
Storage Condition	} Magnesium Oxide
Chemical Incompatibility.	}
Medicinal and Pharmaceutical Uses.	}

5. MAGNESIUM TRISILICATE, $2MgO,3SiO_2,nH_2O$

Preparation: Magnesium trisilicate is prepared by slowly running a solution of magnesium sulphate into a solution of sodium silicate. The precipitated magnesium trisilicate is washed free from sulphate, dried and powdered.

Physical and Chemical Properties: Magnesium trisilicate is a fine, white, odourless and tasteless powder. It is free from grittiness and is slightly hygroscopic. It is practically insoluble in water.

Magnesium trisilicate when treated with any acid such as dilute hydrochloric acid forms magnesium chloride and gelatinous trisilicic acid.

$$Mg_2Si_3O_8 + 4HCl \longrightarrow 2MgCl_2 + H_4Si_3O_8$$
(or $2MgO, 3SiO_2$) Trisilicic acid
(Magnesium trisilicate)

The same reaction takes place when magnesium trisilicate comes into contact with hydrochloric acid in the stomach. It is estimated that one gram of magnesium trisilicate neutralizes about 155 ml of N/10 or 0.1 N hydrochloric acid. A gelatinous mass which is formed covers and protects the ulcer tissue for several hours. The I.P.1985 gives a test for acid absorption which is a measure of its acid neutralizing capacity.

Official Test for Identity: A small quantity is boiled with sodium hydroxide solution and filtered. The filtrate is acidified with dilute hydrochloric acid and boiled. The white gelatinous precipitate that is produced is dissolved in dilute hydrochloric acid and filtered. The filtrate gives the reactions of magnesium (see Chapter 13).

Standard: Magnesium trisilicate contains between 29 per cent and 32 per cent of MgO and between 65 per cent and 68.5 per cent of SiO_2, both calculated with reference to the substance ignited at $1000^{\circ}C$.

Storage Condition: Since it is slightly hygroscopic, store in a well closed container.

Chemical Incompatibility: It is incompatible with acids and forms a gelatinous mass.

Medicinal and Pharmaceutical Uses

Good antacid: It does not produce any rebound acidity like sodium bicarbonate. It does not interfere with peptic digestion.

6. ALUMINIUM HYDROXIDE GEL, Al(OH)₃.

According to I.P.1985, Aluminium Hydroxide Gel is an aqueous suspension of hydrated aluminium oxide together with varying quantities of basic aluminium carbonate and bicarbonate. It may contain glycerin, sorbitol, sucrose or saccharin as sweetening agent and peppermint oil or other flavours. It may also contain suitable antimicrobial agents. 0.5% sodium benzoate or benzoic acid may be used as preservative.

Preparation: For preparing this, a hot solution of potash alum is added slowly to a hot solution of sodium carbonate and not vice versa. The precipitate of aluminium hydroxide is washed thoroughly with hot water till it is found to be free of sulphate. The gel is then adjusted to the required volume with distilled water.

$$3Na_2CO_3 + 2KAl(SO_4)_2 + 3H_2O \longrightarrow 3Na_2SO_4 + K_2SO_4$$
$$\text{Potash alum} \qquad\qquad + 2Al(OH)_3\downarrow + 3CO_2\uparrow$$

If sodium carbonate solution is added to potash alum solution, then it is difficult to wash out the sulphate completely. Due to adsorption by aluminium hydroxide, some carbonate may be present.

Physical and Chemical Properties

Aluminium hydroxide gel is a white viscous suspension which is translucent (that is, allows the light to pass through partially). Small amounts of clear liquid may separate from this on standing. It is insoluble in water and readily soluble in acids and alkalis.

It is amphoteric in nature. It affects both blue litmus and red litmus. Heated strongly, it decomposes into aluminium oxide and water. It reacts with hydrochloric acid to form aluminium chloride.

$$Al(OH)_3 + 3HCl \longrightarrow AlCl_3 + 3H_2O$$

So aluminium hydroxide gel is able to neutralize the acid in the stomach and is a good antacid. It is official in I.P. There is a test for neutralizing capacity prescribed in the I.P.

Official Tests for Identity

A solution in dilute hydrochloric acid gives the reactions of aluminium (see Chapter 13).

Standard: It contains between 3.5 per cent and 4.4 per cent w/w of Al_2O_3.

Storage Condition: Store in tightly closed containers in a cool place and avoid freezing.

Chemical Incompatibility: It is conceivable that aluminium hydroxide gel may be used only in combination with other antacids like magnesium hydroxide or magnesium trisilicate. Under these circumstances no particular incompatibility is envisaged.

Medicinal and Pharmaceutical Uses

Antacid. It is used as an antacid and protective in treating peptic ulcers. It is also used in cases of acute hyperacidity.

7. ALUMINIUM PHOSPHATE, $AlPO_4$

It consists mainly of about 80% of hydrated aluminium orthophosphate.

Preparation

A solution of dried dibasic sodium phosphate in water is added slowly to solution of aluminium chloride and aluminium phosphate is formed along with sodium chloride and hydrochloric acid.

$$AlCl_3.6H_2O + Na_2HPO_4 \longrightarrow AlPO_4\downarrow + 2NaCl + HCl + 6H_2O$$

The hydrochloric acid formed is neutralized by adding diluted ammonia.

$$HCl + NH_4OH \longrightarrow NH_4Cl + H_2O$$

The mixture is then filtered and washed with water to free it from soluble salts such as sodium chloride and ammonium chloride. Then sufficient water is added to get a gel with a concentration of about 4% of aluminium phosphate. Alternatively all the water is removed and the product is dried under suitable conditions to get the dried aluminium phosphate.

Physical and Chemical Properties

Dried aluminium phosphate is a white amorphous powder containing some friable aggregates. It is practically insoluble in water and alcohol but is readily soluble in mineral acids. It is insoluble in solutions of alkali hydroxides.

Aluminium phosphate answers all the reactions of the aluminium ion and the phosphate radical. For this it must be dissolved in nitric acid (for testing for phosphate) and in hydrochloric acid (for testing for aluminium).

Tests for Identity

(1) A solution of aluminium phosphate in hydrochloric acid gives the reactions of aluminium. (See Chapter 13).

(2) A solution of aluminium phosphate in nitric acid gives the reactions of phosphates (see Chapter 13).

Medicinal Use: Antacid

Aluminium phosphate gel, which contains about 4% of aluminium phosphate, is normally used as the antacid. Sweetening agents such as glycerin, sugar or saccharin may be added to make the gel more palatable and oil of peppermint to give a nice flavour. Dried aluminium phosphate tablets (500 mg) are also available flavoured with peppermint. Sodium benzoate or benzoic acid (0.5%) is usually added to the gel to serve as a preservative.

Aluminium phosphate is a slow-acting antacid. It is better than aluminium hydroxide gel in the sense that it does not interfere with the absorption of phosphates from the intestine.

COMBINATIONS OF ANTACIDS

There are three complications usually seen when antacids are used. First, many antacids exert an action on the bowel. For example some have a mild laxative effect (eg. magnesium hydroxide) and some are constipating (eg. aluminium hydroxide). Secondly if the cation (the metallic ion) is absorbed, systemic alkalosis (a condition in which the alkalinity of body fluids and tissues is abnormally high) may be produced (eg. sodium bicarbonate).   Calcium ions may produce hypercalcaemia (the presence in the blood of an abnormally high concentration of calcium). Magnesium and aluminium cause precipitation of phosphate in the gastrointestinal tract and depletion of phosphorus. Finally antacids may affect the absorption of other drugs which may be administered along with antacids such as antichlolinergics and antibiotics. These drugs may be adsorbed by the antacids. Antacids may also alter the pH of the gastric contents thereby delaying the absorption of weak acids and speeding the absorption of basic drugs.

If dyspepsia (indigestion) leading to gas formation in the gut is present, use of a drug like methylpolysiloxane (dimethicone or simethicone) is necessary. Therefore because of the defects associated with the antacids as discussed in the previous paragraph, it is apparent that it is wiser to use a combination of antacids so that the defects can be minimized. For example magnesium hydroxide and aluminium hydroxide may be combined to balance the constipating effect of the latter with the laxative effect of the former. On this basis the following combinations are in regular clinical use:

1. Magnesium and aluminium hydroxides (Magaldrate).

2. Magnesium and aluminium hydroxides, dimethicone (Dioval Forte Tabs),

3. Magnesium and aluminium hydroxides, methylpolysiloxane (Gelusil MPS)

4. Aluminium hydroxide gel, magnesium trisilicate (Gelusil)

5. Aluminium hydroxide gel, magnesium hydroxide, magnesium trisilicate (Gelusil M)

6. Mag. hydroxide, dried alu.hydroxide gel, methylpoly-siloxane, sod. carboxymethyl cellulose (Digene gel).

C. PROTECTIVES AND ADSORBENTS

Protectives and adsorbents are drugs which adsorb intestinal toxins, bacteria etc. and also give a protective coating to the inflamed mucosal walls

1. BISMUTH SUBCARBONATE, $(BiO)_2CO_3$.

Preparation: A solution of normal bismuth nitrate is added with continuous stirring to a warm solution of sodium carbonate. The precipitated bismuth subcarbonate is washed with cold water and dried at a temperature below $60^{\circ}C$. Repeated washing should be avoided as the subcarbonate will decompose to hydroxide.

$$2Bi(NO_3)_3 + 3Na_2CO_3 \longrightarrow (BiO)_2CO_3 + 6NaNO_3 + 2CO_2\uparrow$$

Physical and Chemical Properties

Bismuth subcarbonate is a white, amorphous powder without odour and taste. It is practically insoluble in water and alcohol. It is soluble with effervescence in acids. It is stable in air but is slowly affected by light.

When ignited, it decomposes into yellow bismuth trioxide and carbon dioxide.

$$(BiO)_2CO_3 \xrightarrow{\Delta} Bi_2O_3 + CO_2\uparrow$$

It reacts with acids giving effervescence. The corresponding salt formed is hydrolyzed to the basic salt.

$$(BiO)_2CO_3 + 6HCl \longrightarrow 2BiCl_3 + CO_2\uparrow + 3H_2O$$

$$BiCl_3 + 4H_2O \longrightarrow Bi(OH)_2Cl + 2H_3O^+ + 2Cl^-$$

When hydrogen sulphide is passed through an acidified solution of bismuth subcarbonate, a brownish-black precipitate of bismuth sulphide is obtained. This test is used for group analysis of bismuth.

It is official in B.P.1988.

Official Tests for Identity

Gives the reactions of bismuth and carbonates (see Chapter 13).

Standard: Bismuth subcarbonate contains between 80 and 82.5 percent of Bi, calculated with reference to the dried substance.

Storage Condition: Since bismuth subcarbonate is affected by light, it should be protected from light during storage. So store in an amber coloured bottle in a dark place.

Chemical Incompatibility: Bismuth subcarbonate reacts with acids giving effervescence. Even though it goes into solution forming the corresponding acid salt, the same gets hydrolyzed to the basic salt which is insoluble and indiffusible.

Medicinal Uses. Protective and Adsorbent: It is used as a protective, mild astringent, dusting powder and antiseptic. It finds use in gastric disorders, diarrhoea, dysentery, ulcers, ulcerative colitis etc. It may also be used as an antacid.

2. KAOLIN, Al_2O_3, $2SiO_2$, $2H_2O$.

Preparation: Kaolin occurs in special types of clay known as kaolinite, dickite and nacrite. Heavy kaolin is prepared from these by a process of elutriation.

Physical and Chemical Properties

There are two types of kaolin, heavy and light. Kaolin consists mainly of purified natural, hydrated aluminium silicate, Al_2O_3, $2SiO_2$, $2H_2O$ with traces of magnesium, calcium and iron.

Light kaolin is prepared from kaolin by freeing it from gritty particles by a process of elutriation.

Light kaolin is chemically inert since it is insoluble in all the common solvents. It is official in I.P. There are tests for coarse particles and fine particles prescribed in the I.P. to ensure that the official compound will contain only the fine particles. This is necessary in view of the fact that light kaolin is used as an antidiarrhoeal agent and presence of coarse particles will harm the inflamed mucosal surface of the gut in diarrhoea.

Storage Condition: Store in well-closed containers.

Medicinal Use: Adsorbent (in the treatment of diarrhoea): It is used both for its adsorptive property and also for its ability to coat the mucosa. It is used in diarrhoea due to food poisoning or due to bacteria. It provides relief by adsorbing gases, toxins and bacteria.

D. SALINE CATHARTICS

Saline cathartics are salts which in small doses produce a laxative effect (that is, faeces are passed without griping) whereas a larger dose produces purgation or catharsis (loose watery faeces passed with griping and abdominal pain).

1. SODIUM POTASSIUM TARTRATE, $C_4H_4O_6NaK,4H_2O$

Sodium potassium tartrate is also known as **Rochelle salt**.

Preparation: It is prepared by suspending potassium hydrogen tartrate in boiling water and slowly running in a concentrated solution of sodium carbonate till the solution is neutral to litmus. Then the solution is filtered and evaporated to crystallization.

$$Na_2CO_3 + 2KHC_4H_4O_6 \longrightarrow 2KNaC_4H_4O_6 + CO_2 \uparrow + H_2O.$$
$$\text{Pot.hydrogen} \qquad \text{Sod.pot.tartrate.}$$
$$\text{tartrate}$$

Physical and Chemical Properties

It consists of colourless, rhombic crystals or occurs as a white, crystalline powder. It has no odour and it has a saline, cooling taste. It is very soluble in water. As it effloresces slightly in warm, dry air, the crystals are often coated with a dry powder. When it is strongly heated, it chars giving off inflammable gases and leaves a dark grey, charred residue containing sodium and potassium carbonates. In fact sodium potassium tartrate is assayed by adding N/2 hydrochloric acid to the residue and back titrating the excess of acid with N/2 alkali using methyl orange as indicator.

Tests for Identity

Gives the reactions of sodium, potassium and tartrates (see Chapter 13).

Storage Condition: Since it effloresces in dry air, store in tightly closed containers.

Chemical Incompatibility: Tartrate ion is a sequestering agent. so sodium potassium tartrate is incompatible with metals such as iron and bismuth.

Medicinal Use: Saline Cathartic. Sodium potassium tartrate is used in the form of seidlitz powder which contains 7.5 g of sodium potassium tartrate and 2.5 g each of sodium bicarbonate and tartaric acid, the first two together wrapped in blue paper and the tartaric acid wrapped in white paper. The contents of the two are dissolved in water and the mixture taken while effervescing in a palatable condition.

2. MAGNESIUM SULPHATE, $MgSO_4.7H_2O$ (EPSOM SALTS)

Preparation: It may be prepared by any one of the following methods:

By neutralizing hot, dilute sulphuric acid with magnesium or magnesium oxide or magnesium carbonate.

$$MgO + H_2SO_4 \longrightarrow MgSO_4 + H_2O.$$

Physical and Chemical Properties

Magnesium sulphate occurs in small, colourless needle-like crystals or rhombic prisms without odour and with a cooling saline and bitter taste. It is efflorescent in warm, dry air. When gently heated, it readily loses some of its water of hydration. It becomes completely anhydrous at $200^{\circ}C$. Magnesium sulphate crystallizes from cold water in needles ($MgSO_4.7H_2O$). With many other sulphates, magnesium sulphate forms double salts. They are isomorphous with one another. These double salts have the general formula $M_2SO_4.MgSO_4.6H_2O$ where M represents sodium, potassium, ammonium etc. It is soluble 1 in 1 in water and sparingly soluble in alcohol. It dissolves slowly in 1 part of glycerin. It loses 51.1 percent of its weight when dried. This is due to the loss of all water molecules.

Aqueous solution of magnesium sulphate is neutral to litmus. All the reactions of magnesium and sulphate are answered. Magnesium is precipitated as magnesium ammonium phosphate by the addition of ammonium phosphate in the presence of ammonia. The magnesium ammonium phosphate precipitate ($MgNH_4PO_4$) may be collected, dried and ignited when magnesium pyrophosphate is formed.

$$2MgNH_4PO_4 \longrightarrow Mg_2P_2O_7 + 2NH_3 + H_2O.$$
$$\text{Magnesium}$$
$$\text{pyrophosphate.}$$

This was the previous gravimetric assay method for magnesium sulphate. The magnesium pyrophosphate is collected, dried and weighed.

It is official in I.P.

Official Tests for Identity: Gives reactions characteristic of magnesium and of sulphates (refer Chapter 13).

Standard: Contains not less than 99.0 per cent and not more than the equivalent of 100.0 percent of $MgSO_4$, calculated with reference to the substance ignited (and dried to constant weight at $450^{\circ}C$). (Please note that the content is given in terms of the anhydrous substance).

Storage Condition: It is efflorescent; store in a well-closed container.

Chemical Incompatibility: Magnesium sulphate is incompatible with alkalis forming magnesium hydroxide as precipitate. It is also incompatible with sodium bicarbonate. The magnesium bicarbonate first formed decomposes to the carbonate evolving carbon dioxide.

Assay: This is a complexometric assay. An accurately weighted quantity is dissolved in water. Ammonia-ammonium chloride buffer is added and the mixture is titrated with M/20 disodium ethylenediaminetetraacetate (EDTA or disodium salt of ethylenediaminetetraacetic acid or sodium edetate) using mordant black as indicator.

The buffer of strong ammonia-ammonium chloride solution is added to raise and maintain the pH of the solution at 10, because at this pH only complexation takes place. Magnesium is fixed as unionisable Magnesium – EDTA complex by the EDTA. No blank titration is necessary as in the case of calcium assay. The end point is the appearance of blue colour. The complexation of magenesium by EDTA is given below:

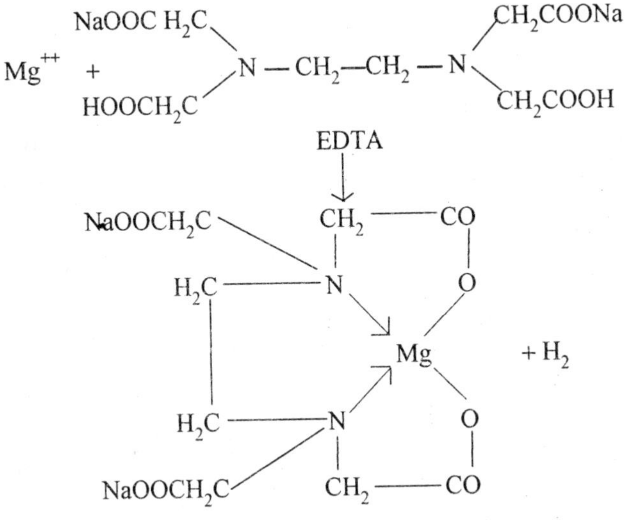

$$Mg^{++} + \underset{\text{HOOCH}_2\text{C}}{\overset{\text{NaOOC H}_2\text{C}}{>}}N-CH_2-CH_2-N\underset{\text{CH}_2\text{COOH}}{\overset{\text{CH}_2\text{COONa}}{<}}$$

EDTA

$\downarrow$

Magnesium - EDTA Complex

Medicinal Use

Cathartic (drastic purgative): This salt is popularly used as a saline cathartic. Both the sulphate and the magnesium ion are not readily absorbed. Therefore water is retained in the intestine. Because of this the quantity and fluidity of the intestinal contents are increased. This mechanically stimulates peristalsis and the bowels are emptied.

CHAPTER 5

TOPICAL AGENTS

Topical means pertaining to a particular locality or place or simply it means 'local'. Therefore the drugs dealt with in this chapter may be substances which are applied directly on the skin or mucous membrane or any other surface.

A. PROTECTIVES

Protectives are substances which are applied over the skin for protecting it from irritation, injury, inflammation etc. They are used in the form of dusting powder etc.

1. TALC (FRENCH CHALK, PURIFIED TALC, TALCUM)
$3MgO, 4SiO_2, H_2O$

Preparation: Purified talc is made by boiling very finely powdered talc with water containing about 2 per cent of hydrochloric acid. The insoluble matter is allowed to settle down and the supernatant liquid is removed. This process is repeated again with more dilute hydrochloric acid. Iron and other soluble impurities are removed by thorough washing with water and the substance is dried at 100°C.

Properties: Talc is a very fine white, or greyish white crystalline powder. It is unctuous, sticking readily to the skin. It is also known as soapstone because it is very soft and greasy to touch like the soap. The specific gravity is 2.6 to 2.8.

Talc is without odour and taste and is insoluble in water. It is insoluble also in dilute acids and alkali hydroxides. Talc is not a good absorbent. Because of this property talc can be used for clarifying solutions of alkaloids, dyes, etc.

Chemically talc is hydrated magnesium silicate with the formula $3MgO, 4SiO_2, H_2O$. It may be considered as a salt of dimetasilicic acid $Mg_3H_2 (Si_2O_6)_2$. It should contain about 31 per cent of MgO and 63.5 per cent of SiO_2 according to this formula but usually there are wide variations.

Talc is an inert magnesium polysilicate not affected by acids or bases and so is useful as a filtering aid and diluent. On fusing with sodium and potassium carbonates, the magnesium part is converted into magnesium carbonate which can be treated with dilute hydrochloi ' acid to bring it into solution. The silica remains insoluble. This property is used in the official test for identity for talc in the I.P.

Official Tests for Identity

1. The talc is fused with sodium and potassium carbonates in the platinum crucible. The mass is extracted with water and hydrochloric acid is added until the effervescence ceases. Evaporate the mixture to dryness. The silicic acid formed is converted on dehydration into silica which is insoluble in water. It is mixed with a little water and filtered. The filtrate contains magnesium chloride which is identified by conversion into magnesium ammonium phosphate (by adding ammonium chloride, ammonia and sodium phosphate).

2. The silicic acid in the above reaction is collected. It gives the reactions of silicates (see Chapter 13).

Storage Condition: Talc is an inert substance not affected by acids or bases or other chemicals. So store in a well-closed container.

Chemical Incompatibility: No specific chemical incompatibility.

Medicinal and Pharmaceutial Uses: It is used as a filtering and distributing medium in the preparation of aromatic waters etc. It is the main ingredient in talcum powders and dusting powders.

2. ZINC OXIDE, ZnO

Preparation

1. Zinc oxide is prepared on a large scale by burning zinc metal in a current of air.

$$2Zn + O_2 \longrightarrow 2ZnO$$

2. In this method, zinc carbonate is prepared first by reacting zinc sulphate with a boiling solution of sodium carbonate. The precipitated basic carbonate of zinc is collected, washed to

remove sulphate, dried and finally gently ignited. It loses carbon dioxide and water, leaving zinc oxide as the residue.

$$2ZnCO_3 . 2Zn(OH)_2 \xrightarrow{\Delta} 4ZnO + 2CO_2 + 3H_2O$$
Basic zinc carbonate.

Properties: Zinc oxide is a very fine white or yellowish white, amorphous powder without gritty particles. It is tasteless and odourless. It gradually absorbs carbon dioxide from the air and is converted into a basic carbonate. It is insoluble in water and alcohol but is soluble in dilute acids, ammonia, ammonium carbonate and alkali hydroxides. Low commerical grades may contain arsenic and lead as impurities and therefore are unsuitable for medicinal use.

As already stated, it readily dissolves in acids, ammonia and ammonium carbonate solution, it forms zinc chloride with hydrochloric acid and the corresponding zinc ammonium salt with ammonia and ammonium carbonate.

$$ZnO + 2HCl \longrightarrow ZnCl_2 + H_2O$$

$$ZnO + 4NH_4OH \longrightarrow Zn(NH_3)_4(OH)_2 + 3H_2O$$

$$ZnO + 2(NH_4)_2CO_3 \longrightarrow Zn(NH_3)_4(OH)_2 + 2CO_2\uparrow + H_2O$$

It is official in I.P.

Official Tests for Identity

1. When strongly heated, zinc oxide gets a yellow colour which disappears on cooling.

2. A solution in dilute hydrochloric acid, after neutralization of the excess acid, gives the reactions characteristic of zinc (see Chapter 13).

Standard: Contains not less than 99 per cent and not more than the equivalent of 100.5 per cent of ZnO, calculated with reference to the substance ignited to constant weight.

Storage Condition: Since it absorbs carbon dioxide from the air, store it in a well-closed container.

Assay: An accurately weighed quantity of the substance and a specific quantity of ammonium chloride are dissolved in a known excess of N/1 sulphuric acid with the aid of gentle heat, if necessary. When solution is complete, it is titrated against N/1 sodium hydroxide using methyl orange as indicator. Appearance of yellow colour is the end point.

The zinc oxide reacts with the sulphuric acid and the excess of acid left after the reaction is titrated against the alkali. Ammonium chloride is added to prevent a poor end point due to precipitation of zinc hydroxide during the course of the titration and at the end point.

$$ZnO + H_2SO_4 \longrightarrow ZnSO_4 + H_2O$$

$$H_2SO_4 + 2NaOH \longrightarrow Na_2SO_4 + 2H_2O$$

Medicinal Use. Astringent and topical protective: Zinc oxide is a mild antiseptic and astringent. In the form of zinc oxide ointment or dusting powder, it is used in the treatment of eczema, ringworm, pruritus and psoriasis. It is also widely used in the manufacture of plasters.

3. CALAMINE

According to B.P. 1988, calamine is basic zinc carbonate suitably coloured with ferric oxide. According to the I.P. 1985, calamine is zinc oxide coloured with ferric oxide. It is an amorphous, reddish brown powder and the colour depends on the variety and amount of ferric oxide present and the method by which it is incorporated. It is practically insoluble in water and completely soluble in mineral acids. Since there is a possibility of adulteration with dyes, there are tests for water soluble dyes and alcohol soluble dyes.

Official Tests for identity (I.P)

1. A specified quantity is shaken with dilute hydrochloric acid and filtered. The filtrate gives the reactions of zinc (see Chapter 13).

2. A little quantity is mixed with dilute hydrochloric acid, heated to boiling and filtered. To the filtrate is added ammonium thiocyanate solution. A reddish colour is produced.

Standard: Contains between 98 and 100.5 percent of ZnO, calculated with reference to the ignited substance.

Storage Condition: Store in well-closed containers.

Medicinal and Pharmaceutical Uses. Topical Protective: Widely used in lotions, oinments and dusting powders as a soothing agent. It is used in sunburn, eczema and urticaria and some other skin conditions. Calamine lotion (Lotio Calaminae) is very popular.

4. ZINC STEARATE, $(C_{17}H_{35}COO)_2 Zn$

Zinc stearate is a mixture of zinc salts obtained from commercial stearic acid which itself is prepared from the hydrolysis of fats. It consists mainly of variable proportions of zinc stearate and zinc palmitate.

Preparation: Stearic acid is added slowly with constant stirring to a hot solution of sodium carbonate. Then the mixture is cooled and zinc acetate or zinc sulphate is added to the sodium stearate formed. Zinc stearate is precipitated. It is collected, washed and dried.

$$Na_2CO_3 + 2C_{17}H_{35}COOH \longrightarrow 2C_{17}H_{35}COONa + CO_2\uparrow$$
$$+ H_2O$$
$$2C_{17}H_{35}COONa + ZnSO_4 \longrightarrow (C_{17}H_{35}COO)_2 Zn + Na_2SO_4$$

Physical and Chemical Properties

Zinc stearate is a fine, white, bulky powder, free from grittiness with a faint but characteristic odour. It is unctuous to touch and readily sticks to the skin. It is practically insoluble in water.

When it is heated at a high temperature, it fuses and gives fumes which are inflammable and have smell of burning fat. A residue of zinc oxide is left behind. It is decomposed by hot mineral acids with liberation of stearic and palmitic acids.

$$(C_{17}H_{35}COO)_2 Zn + 2HCl \longrightarrow 2C_{17}H_{35}COOH + ZnCl_2$$
$$\text{Stearic acid}$$

It is official in I.P.

Official Tests for Identity

1. To a small quantity of the substance, hydrochloric acid is added and boiled. An oily layer is produced on the surface. The lower aqueous layer, after neutralisation, gives the reactions of zinc (see Chapter 13).

2. The oily upper layer obtained in the above test is separated and washed with boiling water. It is cooled and dried at 105°C. The melted acid solidifies at a temperature below 54°C.

In this test stearic acid is produced in test (1). This is collected, washed and dried. It is allowed to solidify. Since zinc stearate is a mixture of zinc salts of stearic and other acids, mainly palmitic acid, it is possible that the solidification temperature may be lower than 54°C, if it contains more of other acids. So this test is to control the amount of other fatty acid salts of zinc other than zinc stearate present in the sample.

Standard: Zinc stearate contains between 12.5 and 14.5 per cent of ZnO.

Storage Condition: Store in well-closed containers

Chemical Incompatibility: It is incompatible with mineral acids. Since it is a divalent soap, it is also incompatible with monovalent salts and alkalis.

Medicinal and Pharmaceutical Uses

Dusting Powder: Since zinc stearate is a mild antiseptic and astringent, it is used in the form of dusting powder or ointment in several skin conditions. Sometimes it is used as a solid diluent.

5. TITANIUM DIOXIDE, TiO_2

Titanium dioxide occurs in nature in the minerals rutile, brookite and ilmenite. Magnetic iron ores usually contain titanium.

Preparation: Titanium dioxide is prepared by heating ilmenite ($FeTiO_3$) with hydrogen chloride and chlorine.

$$2FeTiO_3 + 4HCl + Cl_2 \longrightarrow 2FeCl_3 + 2\,TiO_2 + 2H_2O.$$

Physical and Chemical Properties

Titanium dioxide is a white or almost white amorphous infusible powder. It is odourless and tasteless. It is insoluble in water and in dilute mineral acids. It is slowly soluble in hot concentrated sulphuric acid. Because of the high refractive index (2.7), titanium dioxide has great opacity.

It dissolves in hydrofluoric acid also. It is reduced to titanium metal when it is heated with carbon, calcium, sodium or magnesium. Titanium dioxide in dilute sulphuric acid reacts with hydrogen peroxide and gives an orange red colour. This is due to the formation of titanium peroxide and this test is used as a test for identity for titanium dioxide.

It is official in I.P.

Official Tests for Identity

1. A small quantity is dissolved in concentrated sulphuric acid containing a little sodium sulphate with the aid of heat and diluted. To this solution is added strong hydrogen peroxide solution. An orange-red colour is produced.

2. To another quantity of solution obtained in (1) granulated zinc is added. A violet blue colour is produced after forty five minutes.

Standard: Contains not less than 98 percent of TiO_2, caluculated with reference to the dried substance.

Storage Condition: Store in well-closed containers made of glass or any metal other than aluminium.

Chemical Incompatibility: Incompatible with reducing agents.

Medicinal and Pharmaceutical Uses

Pharmaceutical aid and topical protective: Since it spreads well, it is used as a white pigment in paints. Because of its high refractive index it is used in sun-tan preparations.

6. SILICONE POLYMERS

Compounds that are formed as a result of the bonding of silicon, oxygen and carbon by condensation are known as silicones. One of the building blocks of silicones is dimethyldihydroxysilane, $(CH_3)_2Si$ $(OH)_2$.

Two dimethyldihydroxysilane molecules undergo condensation with elimination of a molecule of water. Repeated condensation of thse molecules results in the formation of macro molecules (big molecules) or polymers. These are known as *silicones*. The Si-O-Si linkage in these molecules is very strong.

The general formula of silicones may be given as $[(CH_3)_2SiO-]n$. Silicones obtained by starting with dimethyldihydroxysilane are known as *silicone oils*.

The silicones are stable at very high and very low temperatures and are water repellent. Silicones are used for making water-proof cloth and lubricants which do not feeeze even at very low temperatures. Activated dimethicone is official in I.P.

ACTIVATED DIMETHICONE

Activated dimethicone is activated polydimethylsiloxane. It is also known as simethicone. It has the formula $(CH_3)_3Si - [OSi(CH_3)_2]$ $- CH_3$.

Preparation: It is prepared by the hydrolysis and polycondensation of dichlorodimethylsilane, $(CH_3)_2SiCl_2$ and chlorotrimethylsilane, $(CH_3)_3SiCl$.

Properties: It is a translucent (partly opaque and partly transparent), grey, viscous liquid. It is almost odourless and tasteless. It is insoluble in water and in alcohol.

Official Test for Identity: The sample is treated with carbon tetrachloride and dilute hydrochloric acid and shaken well for five minutes. The lower layer is shaken with anhydrous sodium sulphate to remove any water. The mixture is centrifuged till a clear supernatant liquid is obtained. The infra-red absorption spectrum of the resulting solution exhibits maxima at the same wavelengths as in the spectrum of a solution of polydimethylsiloxane R.S. (Reference Standard).

Standard: It contains not less than 90 per cent of polydimethyl-siloxane, [(CH$_3$)$_2$SiO-]n.

Storage Condition: Store in tightly closed containers.

Medicinal and Pharmaceutical Uses

Protective and Defoaming Agent: Dimethicone is used for preparing dimethicone cream (formerly official in B.P.C.). This cream is used to protect the skin against colostomy and other discharges and to prevent bed sores and napkin-rash. (Colostomy is an operation to make an artificial opening so that the colon opens on to the anterior abdominal wall. This operation is done when there is an obstruction in the colon). Dimethicone is also included in antacid mixtures to treat cases of flatulence.

B. ANTIMICROBIALS AND ASTRINGENTS

Antimicrobials are drugs which destroy the microorganisms. They can be divided into disinfectants and antiseptics. A disinfectant or germicide is a chemical which destroys microorganisms by killing them. Spores of the microorganisms are not usually killed by disinfectants. Disinfectants can also be more specifically called as bactericides, fungicides, virucides, amoebicicdes etc. depending on whether they are able to kill bacteria, fungi, viruses, amoebae etc. respectively. They can be used for the (external) sterilization of instruments, articles, surfaces, rooms etc. Sterilization is the total elimination of all kinds of microorganisms including their spores and the product thus obtained is said to be sterile. An antiseptic is a substance which eliminates the microorganisms by inhibiting their growth. They can be safely applied to the skin or mucous membrane to prevent sepsis.

An astringent is a drug which makes the cells shrink by precipitating proteins from their surfaces. They are used in lotions to harden and protect the skin and to reduce bleeding from minor abrasions. Other preparations in which they are used are antiperspirant preparations, mouth washes, eye drops, throat lozenges etc. Many of the drugs discussed below possess both antimicrobial and astringent properties.

1. HYDROGEN PEROXIDE, H_2O_2

Hydrogen peroxide was discovered by L.J.Thenard in 1818 and he designated it as "Oxygenated Water". Hydrogen peroxide solution is official in I.P.

Preparation:

The methods for commercial manufacture may be divided into two groups:

(a) the non-electrolytic and (b) the electrolytic.

(a) The Non-electrolytic Methods

1. Barium peroxide is made into a thin cream with water. It is added slowly with constant stirring to dilute sulphuric acid, which should be kept cooled in ice:

$$BaO_2 + H_2SO_4 \longrightarrow BaSO_4\downarrow + H_2O_2.$$

2. Hydrogen peroxide can also be made by decomposing barium peroxide with phosphoric acid, or by passing carbon dioxide through a suspension of barium peroxide in water:

$$3BaO_2.8H_2O + 2\,H_3PO_4 \longrightarrow Ba_3(PO_4)_2\downarrow + 3H_2O_2 + 24H_2O$$

3. Another method is by decomposition of sodium peroxide with sulphuric acid at a low temperature ($-2°C$). Most of the sodium sulphate produced is crystallised as the decahydrate, $Na_2SO_4.10H_2O$) and the hydrogen peroxide is subsequently distilled under 20 mm, pressure:

$$Na_2O_2 + H_2SO_4 \longrightarrow H_2O_2 + Na_2SO_4$$

(b) The Electrolytic Methods

1. Hydrogen peroxide is prepared by electrolysis of sulphuric acid to peroxydisulphuric acid which is hydrolysed to give the product. In this electrolysis, sulphuric acid is oxidised to peroxydisulphuric acid ($H_2S_2O_8$).

$$2H_2SO_4 \longrightarrow H_2S_2O_8 + H_2.$$

Peroxydisulphuric acid, when heated, forms peroxysulphuric acid, H_2SO_5 (Caro's acid).

$$H_2S_2O_8 + H_2O \xrightarrow{\Delta} H_2SO_5 + H_2SO_4$$

The peroxysulphuric acid is then hydrolysed by further heating to give hydrogen peroxide.

$$H_2SO_5 + H_2O \longrightarrow H_2O_2 + H_2SO_4.$$

2. By a modification of this method, a solution of ammonium sulphate and sulphuric acid is electrolysed to form ammonium peroxydisulphate:

$$(NH_4)_2SO_4 + H_2SO_4 \longrightarrow 2NH_4HSO_4.$$

$$2NH_4HSO_4 \longrightarrow (NH_4)_2S_2O_8 + H_2$$

Hydrogen peroxide may be distilled directly from the ammonium peroxydisulphate solution:

$$(NH_4)_2S_2O_8 + 2H_2O \longrightarrow 2NH_4HSO_4 + H_2O_2.$$

All these procedures, both non-electrolytic and electrolytic, produce a solution of hydrogen peroxide which may be concentrated by distillation under reduced pressure to produce a concentration of even upto 90 per cent H_2O_2.

Physical and Chemical Properties: Hydrogen peroxide is stable in solutions of high purity. However, it decomposes rapidly in alkaline solutions or under catalytic influences, such as copper, iron or manganese ions:

$$2H_2O_2 \longrightarrow 2H_2O + O_2\uparrow$$

When pure, hydrogen peroxide decomposes very slowly. Its stability is increased by making it slightly acid (eg. by adding sulphuric or phosphoric acid) and also by adding very small quantities of preservatives or stabilizers such as boric acid, urea, acetanilide or hexamine (not more than 0.025 per cent).

Hydrogen peroxide in aqueous solution ionizes to give the peroxide ion.

$$H_2O_2 \rightleftarrows 2H^+ + O_2^{2-}$$

Potassium permanganate in acid solution is rapidly reduced. Here hydrogen peroxide acts as a reducing agent.

$$2KMnO_4 + 3H_2SO_4 + 5H_2O_2 \longrightarrow K_2SO_4 + 2MnSO_4 + 8H_2O + 5O_2\uparrow$$

Oxygen is always produced when hydrogen peroxide functions as a reducing agent.

The official solution is 6 per cent w/v i.e. it is 20 volumes hydrogen peroxide which means it will give 20 times its volume of oxygen on heating.

Official Tests for Identity:

1. Decomposes with effervescence when made alkaline and heated, evolving oxygen.

2. To a small quantity mixed with dilute sulphuric acid, add potassium chromate and solvent ether. The ethereal layer is coloured blue (the blue colour is due to a perchromic acid which is more soluble in ether. This test is capable of detecting hydrogen peroxide as dilute as 0.0015%).

Standard. Hydrogen peroxide solution contains between 5 per cent and 7 per cent w/v of H_2O_2 corresponding to about 20 times its volume of available oxygen.

Storage Condition. Hydrogen peroxide solution should be stored only in a glass stoppered bottle and cork, rubber or metal should not be used for storing it, as it will attack them. Plastic protected metal caps may be used as stoppers. Store in light resistant containers in a cool place. It should not be stored for long periods.

Chemical Incompatibility: Hydrogen peroxide functions as an active oxidizing agent and so is incompatible with sulphides and sulphites (oxidized to sulphates), arsenites (oxidized to arsenates) and ferrous salts (oxidized to ferric salts). It also acts as a reducing agent and in that sense is incompatible with substances like potassium permanganate.

Assay: It is acidified with dilute sulphuric acid and titrated against N/10 potassium permanganate.

$$2KMnO_4 + 3H_2SO_4 + 5H_2O_2 \longrightarrow K_2SO_4 + 2MnSO_4$$
$$+ 8H_2O + 5O_2\uparrow$$

or $O+H_2O_2 \longrightarrow H_2O + O_2\uparrow$

Medicinal and Pharmaceutical Use: As an antiseptic and topical anti-infective: It is especially useful in cleaning wounds specially where pus is present.

2. POTASSIUM PERMANGANATE, KMnO$_4$

Preparation: Manganese dioxide is fused with excess of potassium hydroxide in the presence of a free supply of air, or in the presence of an oxidizing agent such as potassium chlorate:

$$6KOH + 3MnO_2 + KClO_3 \longrightarrow 3K_2MnO_4 + KCl + 3H_2O$$

	Manganese	Potassium	Potassium
	dioxide	chlorate	manganate

The green residue consisting of potassium manganate is extracted with water. From this potassium permanganate is made by any one of the following three methods:

1. By passing carbon dioxide. Two-thirds of the manganate are converted into potassium permanganate while the one-third is precipitated as manganese dioxide:

$$3K_2MnO_4 + 2CO_2 \longrightarrow 2KMnO_4 + MnO_2 + 2K_2CO_3$$

2. All the manganate may be converted into permanganate by passing chlorine through the solution.

$$2K_2MnO_4+Cl_2 \longrightarrow 2KMnO_4 + 2KCl$$

3. By electrolysing a warm solution of the manganate.

$$2K_2MnO_4 + 2H_2O \longrightarrow KMnO_4 + 2KOH + H_2\uparrow$$

The solution obtained by any one of the above methods is filtered and concentrated until potassium permanganate separates as crystals.

Physical Properties: Potassium permanganate occurs in the form of slender, dark purple, monoclinic prisms, almost opaque by transmitted light and having a blue metallic lustre by reflected light. It has a solubility of 1 in 15 in water. It is reduced by alcohol.

Chemical Properties: Potassium permanganate is a very powerful oxidizing agent when dry and also in solution. Explosions may occur when it comes into contact with organic or other readily oxidizable material such as cork or charcoal. When mixed with glycerin, it burns.

Potassium permanganate acts as an oxidizing agent because it is able to produce nascent oxygen in solution.

$$2KMnO_4 + 3H_2SO_4 \longrightarrow K_2SO_4 + 2MnSO_4 + 3H_2O + 5(O)$$
$$\text{(acid solution)}$$

$$2KMnO_4 + H_2O \longrightarrow 2MnO_2 + 2KOH + 3(O)$$
$$\text{(alkaline or neutral solution)}$$

1. Hydrogen peroxide decolourises acidified potassium permanaganate.

$$2KMnO_4 + 3H_2SO_4 + 5H_2O_2 \longrightarrow K_2SO_4 + 2MnSO_4 + 8H_2O + 5O_2\uparrow$$

2. It is also decolourised by oxalic acid in sulphuric acid in the hot condition.

$$5H_2C_2O_4 \cdot 2H_2O + 2KMnO_4 + 3H_2SO_4 \longrightarrow K_2SO_4 + 2MnSO_4 + 18H_2O + 10CO_2\uparrow$$
Oxalic acid

3. On heating potassium permanganate at 240°C, very pure oxygen is evolved and a black powdery residue of potassium manganate and manganese dioxide is left.

$$2KMnO_4 \xrightarrow{\Delta} K_2MnO_4 + MnO_2 + O_2$$
Potassium
manganate

When a little water is added to the residue, potassium permanganate is reformed along with potassium hydroxide.

$$3K_2MnO_4 + 2H_2O \longrightarrow 2KMnO_4 + MnO_2 + 4KOH$$

4. Iodine is liberated from potassium iodide by an acid solution of potassium permanganate.

$$2KMnO_4 + 10KI + 8H_2SO_4 \longrightarrow 6K_2SO_4 + 2MnSO_4 + 5I_2 + 8H_2O.$$

5. Ferrous salts are oxidised to ferric salts by acidified permanganate.

$$2KMnO_4 + 10FeSO_4 + 8H_2SO_4 \longrightarrow K_2SO_4 + 2MnSO_4$$
$$+ 5Fe_2(SO_4)_3 + 8H_2O$$

It is official in I.P.

Official Tests for Identity.

1. A solution in water, acidified with sulphuric acid and heated to 70°C is decolourised by solution of hydrogen peroxide.

2. On strong heating, it evolves oxygen and leaves a black residue. On adding water to the residue, potassium hydroxide solution is formed (reaction No.3 above).

   This after neutralisation with hydrochloric acid, gives the reactions characteristic of potassium (see Chapter 13).

Standard: Contains not less than 99.0 per cent of $KMnO_4$.

Storage Condition: Store in a well-closed container.

Chemical Incompatibility: Potassium permanganate is incompatible with reducing agents and substances liable to be oxidised. Great care should be taken while handling potassium permanganate, since dangerous explosions may occur when it comes into contact with organic or other readily oxidisable substance either in solution or in the dry condition.

Assay: By titration against N/10 oxalic acid. The oxalic acid is acidified with sulphuric acid and kept at 70°C throughout the titration. If the temperature is not maintained at 70°C, the reaction will be slow (refer reaction 2 above).

$$2\ KMnO_4 \longrightarrow 5(O)$$

$$5(O) + 5\ (COOH)_2 \longrightarrow 10CO_2 + 5H_2O$$

The permanganate should be taken in the burette and the end point is appearance of a pale pink colour.

Medicinal or Pharmaceutical Use. As **anti-infective** (i.e. as disinfectant). Its action is due to the liberation of oxygen which oxidizes the protein of the bacteria and kills them. Used as a mouthwash and gargle.

3. BLEACHING POWDER OR CHLORINATED LIME, Ca (OCl) Cl

Chlorinated lime is official in I.P. 1966.

Preparation: Slaked lime is spread upon shelves in a box like container and subjected to the action of chorine gas, which is introduced at the top of the chamber and flows through the contents. The temperature is maintained below 25°C so that formation of calcium chlorate is brought down. When the absorption of chlorine is complete, which may take about 12 to 24 hours, powdered lime is sent into the chamber so that any excess chlorine may be absorbed.

$$Ca(OH)_2 + Cl_2 \longrightarrow Ca(OCl)Cl + H_2O$$

Physical and Chemical Properties: Bleaching powder is a white or grayish white granular powder having a pronounced odour of chlorine. It is considered as consisting of "calcium chloro-hypochlorite", $Ca(OCl)$ Cl, H_2O, which is intermediate between calcium chloride, $CaCl_2$ and calcium hypochlorite, $Ca (OCl)_2$. It has varying amounts of calcium hydroxide and moisture. Although it becomes moist on exposure to air, it is not deliquescent (ie, from the atmosphere). When it is exposed to the air, it slowly decomposes:

$$Ca(OCl) Cl + CO_2 + H_2O \longrightarrow CaCO_3 + HCl + HOCl$$

$$HOCl + HCl \longrightarrow Cl_2 + H_2O$$

and for this reason chlorinated lime should be stored only in tightly stoppered bottles. One may see bleaching powder being used in latrines and other places because chlorine is produced as given above and sterilizes the places. It is used mainly for its disinfecting properties and as a bleaching agent.

Offical Tests for Identity:

1. When hydrochloric acid is added to bleaching powder, chlorine is copiously evolved.

2. Gives the reactions characterisitic of calcium and chlorides (refer Chapter 13).

Standard. Chlorinated Lime is required to contain not less than 30% w/w of available chlorine.

Storage Condition. Refer the reaction with carbon dioxide and moisture. Becuase of this it must be stored in a tightly stoppered container.

Chemical Incompatibility: Chlorinated lime is incompatible with soluble iodides and bromides and mineral acids.

Assay: An aqueous suspension of the substance is first treated with excess of potassium iodide and acetic acid. Acetic acid, like other acids, liberates chlorine from chlorinated lime as below:

$$Ca(OCl)Cl + 2CH_3COOH \longrightarrow (CH_3COO)_2Ca + HOCl + HCl$$

$$HOCl + HCl \longrightarrow Cl_2 + H_2O.$$

The liberated chlorine displaces an equivalent amount of iodine from potassium iodide:

$$2KI + Cl_2 \longrightarrow 2KCl + I_2$$

This iodine is titrated against N/10 sodium thiosulphate using starch mucilage as indicator.

$$2Na_2S_2O_3 + I_2 \longrightarrow Na_2S_4O_6 + 2NaI$$

Medicinal and Pharmaceutical Use : As given under properties.

4. IODINE, I_2

Preparation: Iodine is mostly obtained from sea-weeds, Chile salt petre mother liquors and various brines.

A. From Sea-Weeds: Most sea weeds contain iodine, the largest content (0.5 per cent) in the stem of Laminaria digitata. Others such as Fucus vesiculosis usually contain much less.

Dried sea weed is burnt and the ash or kelp is extracted with water. The extract is concentrated and the less soluble salts such as the sulphates and chlorides of sodium and potassium crystallize and are filtered out. Next sulphuric acid is added and this results in the decomposition of sulphides and thiosulphates with consequent precipitation of sulphur which is removed. The sulphuric acid also converts the iodides and bromides into sulphates. Hydrogen iodide and hydrogen bromide are produced and remain in solution. Then any of the two following procedures may be used.

1. The acid solution which now contains the freely soluble iodides with only small proportions of bromides and chlorides is treated with the correct proportion of chlorine and iodine is precipitated:

$$2HI + Cl_2 \longrightarrow I_2 + 2HCl$$

or

2. The acid solution is warmed in a still and manganese dioxide is added from time to time. The liberated iodine volatilises and is condensed in suitable receivers.

$$2HI + MnO_2 + H_2SO_4 \longrightarrow MnSO_4 + 2H_2O + I_2$$

Iodine obtained by either of these methods may contain iodine chloride, ICl and iodine bromide, IBr. The iodine from these is liberated by sublimation with a small quantity of potassium iodide:

$$ICl + KI \longrightarrow KCl + I_2$$
$$IBr + KI \longrightarrow KBr + I_2$$

This treatment also removes iodine cyanide, which is usually present.

B. From Chile Salt Petre: Crude chile salt petre contains about 0.2 per cent of iodine chiefly in the form of sodium iodate, $NaIO_3$. The mother liquor remaining after the crystallization of sodium nitrate from solution of caliche (crude Chile salt petre) is treated with sodium bisulphite:

$$2NaIO_3 + 5NaHSO_3 \longrightarrow Na_2SO_4 + 3NaHSO_4 + I_2 + H_2O$$

Alternatively the mother liquor is mixed with a stream of sulphur dioxide to liberate the iodine :

$$2NaIO_3 + 4H_2O + 5SO_2 \longrightarrow Na_2SO_4 + 4H_2SO_4 + I_2$$

In both the cases the precipitated iodine is collected and purified by sublimation.

Physical and Chemical Properties:

Iodine is a greyish black solid having a metallic lustre and a characteristic penetrating odour. It crystallizes in large rhombic plates or granules. It is appreciably volatile at ordinary temperatures and should be stored in bottles with glass stoppers. This is because the vapour attacks both cork and rubber. It melts at 114°C, but sublimes at temperatures below its melting point. It gives off a violet-coloured vapour which is one of the heaviest known gases, 8.8 times as heavy as air. The liquid boils at 183°C. It has a specific gravity of 4.93 and is the heaviest nonmetallic element.

Iodine is only very slightly soluble in water, but is more soluble in alcohol. It dissolves easily in ether, chloroform and carbon disulphide. It also dissolves in solutions of potassium iodide forming the compound KI_3.

$$KI + I_2 \rightleftharpoons KI_3$$

The I_{3-} ion is formed by the union of I_2 and an iodide ion (I^-) which is attracted to the iodine molecule by a coordinate covalent bond. Solutions of iodine in chloroform, carbon disulphide and liquid paraffin are violet in colour, i.e. the natural colour of iodine vapour, indicating that the iodine exists as such in solution. However solutions in water, alcohol and aqueous iodides are reddish brown in colour, the reason being probabaly the chemical combination of iodine with the solvent (refer solution of iodine in potassium iodide given above).

Iodine gives with mucilage of starch a deep blue colour. The blue colour disappears on warming but reappears on cooling. This is a very characteristic and sensitive reaction.

Iodine functions as an oxidizing agent. Many reducing agents are oxidised by it and sodium thiosulphate is the most important of them.

$$2Na_2S_2O_3 + I_2 \longrightarrow 2NaI + Na_2S_4O_6$$
Sodium thiosulphate

Ferrous chloride, hydrogen sulphide and sulphurous acid are also oxidised.

$$2FeCl_2 + I_2 + 2HCl \longrightarrow 2HI + 2FeCl_3$$
Ferrous   Ferric
chloride   chloride

$$H_2S + I_2 + H_2O \longrightarrow 2HI + H_2SO_4$$
$$\underset{\text{Sulphurous acid}}{H_2SO_3} + I_2 + H_2O \longrightarrow 2HI + \underset{\text{Sulphuric acid}}{H_2SO_4}$$

Iodine functions also as a reducing agent in the presence of strong oxidising agents like nitric acid which oxidizes it to iodic acid.

$$I_2 + 10HNO_3 \longrightarrow 2\underset{\text{Iodic acid}}{HIO_3} + 10NO_2 + 4H_2O$$

With alkalis, iodine gives the corresponding iodides and iodates on heating.

$$3I_2 + 6NaOH \xrightarrow{\Delta} 5NaI + NaIO_3 + 3H_2O$$

Iodine reacts with iron to convert it to ferrous iodide.

$$Fe + I_2 \longrightarrow FeI_2$$

Iodine is official in I.P.

Tests for Identity

Official

1. When gently heated in a test tube, it gives off violet coloured vapours which condense forming a bluish black crystalline sublimate at the top of the test tube.

2. With solution of potassium iodide and starch, a deep blue colour is produced which disappears on boiling and reappears on cooling.

Non-Official

Iodine is easily reduced by many reducing agents, especially sodium thiosulphate. Iodine is decolourised when a solution of sodium thiosulphate is added to it.

Standard: Iodine contains between 99.5 per cent and 100.5 per cent of I.

Storage Condition: It is appreciably volatile at ordinary temperatures and should be stored in well-closed bottles fitted with glass stoppers or well waxed stoppers.

Chemical Incompatibility: Iodine is incompatible with alkalis, reducing agents and strong oxidising agents.

Assay: Since iodine is volatile, it is weighed in a stoppered bottle. An accurately weighed quantity is dissolved in a solution of potassium iodide and slightly acidified with dil. acetic acid. It is titrated against N/10 sodium thiosulphate using starch mucilage as indicator.

$$2Na_2S_2O_3 + I_2 \longrightarrow Na_2S_4O_6 + 2NaI$$

Medicinal and Pharmaceutical Uses of Iodine:

Disinfectant. Iodine is an effective disinfectant. It acts by oxidizing the protoplasm of organisms. In the presence of organic matter its action is very much reduced.

Iodine when administered orally will be converted to inorganic iodide ion in the gastro-intestinal tract. Its systemic effect is therefore the same as that of a corresponding quantity of inorganic iodide.

Pharmaceutically iodine preparations are usually externally used as antiseptics or internally as a source of iodine for the thyroid gland.

THE IODINE SOLUTIONS

There are three iodine solutions official in I.P.'66.

1. Strong iodine solution.
2. Weak iodine solution.
3. Aqueous iodine solution.

Strong Iodine Solution contains 10% w/v of iodine whereas the content of iodine in Weak Iodine Solution is 2 per cent w/v. The content of iodine in Aqueous Iodine Solution is between these two, viz. 5 per cent w/v. Naturally the amount of potassium iodide in Aqueous Iodine Solution which contains no alcohol is relatively more than in the other two solutions which contain alcohol.

Aqueous Iodine Solution

Also known as Lugol's solution. This is the only official solution of iodine which contains no alcohol. It contains 5.0 per cent w/v of iodine and 10.0 per cent w/v of potassium iodide. In making this solution, potassium iodide may be replaced by sodium iodide.

Strong Iodine Solution

This contains 10.0 per cent w/v of iodine and 6.0 per cent w/v of potassium iodide. Iodine is dissolved in a mixture of potassium iodide solution and alcohol 90 per cent. Potassium iodide may be replaced by sodium iodide.

Assay: For this purpose a 25% v/v dilution with alcohol 90 per cent is prepared.

For Iodine: 20 ml is titrated against N/10 sodium thiosulphate using starch mucilage as indicator.

For Potassium Iodide: 10 ml of the solution is diluted with water, hydrochloric acid and potassium cyanide are added and titrated with M/20 potassium iodate until the dark brown solution becomes pale yellow. Then solution of starch is added and the titration is continud until the blue colour is discharged.

Here the potassium iodate obviously reacts with both the potassium iodide and free iodine. The reactions are given below:

$$KIO_3 + 2KI + 3KCN + 6HCl \longrightarrow 6KCl + 3ICN + 3H_2O$$

$$KIO_3 + 2I_2 + 6HCl \longrightarrow KCl + 5ICl + 3H_2O$$

The volume of M/20 iodate used in reacting with the potassium iodide only is given by subtracting from the total volume half the volume of N/10 thiosulphate. Since the concentration of acid is low, starch can be conveniently used as an indicator.

Weak Iodine Solution: This is also known as Iodine Tincture. This contains 2 per cent of iodine and 2.5 per cent of potassium iodide. It is also assayed in the same way as Strong Solution of Iodine. Potassium iodide may be replaced by sodium iodide.

Assay: For iodine and for potassium iodide as for Strong Solution of Iodine.

Uses: Aqueous Iodine Solution is used as a source of iodine and used internally in cases of thyroid deficiency. The alcoholic solutions are used as antiseptics and disinfectants. Even though the potassium iodide in them is enough to keep the iodine in solution, the alcohol facilitates the antiseptic action by dissolving the cutaneous fat and enabling the iodine to exert its disinfectant action more effectively.

Storage: as for iodine.

POVIDONE – IODINE (P.V.P. – IODINE)

Povidone-iodine belongs to the class of indophores. These are large organic molecules which carry loosely bound iodine. This iodine is liberated slowly at the site of application. The most popular of the indophores is povidone-iodine which is a complex produced by the interaction of iodine and polyvinyl pyrrolidone. This complex contains about 9-12 per cent of available iodine.

Properties: Povidone-iodine is a yellowish brown amorphous powder with a characteristic odour. It is slightly hygroscopic. It is soluble in water and alcohol. The aqueous solution is acidic to litmus. The solution is transparent and reddish brown and it has a faint iodine odour. As the solution is diluted more and more, the free iodine content increases and it becomes more powerfully disinfectant. Therefore povidone-iodine solution should be well diluted before use.

Storage Condition: Since it is slightly hygroscopic and also because it contains volatile free iodine, store in well-closed containers.

Chemical Incompatibility: Since it contains loosely held free iodine, it is incompatible with reducing agents like sodium thiosulphate.

Medicinal Use: Disinfectant. The advantages of povidone-iodine are that it is nonirritating, nontoxic and nonstaining and also exerts prolonged germicidal action. It is used against bacteria and fungi mainly, that is in diseases such as boils, burns, ulcers, furunculosis (occurrence of several boils at the same time and also repeated appearance of boils in the skin over a period of weeks or months), otitis externa (inflammation of the skin of the external ear), tinea (ringworm) and vaginitis (inflammation of the vagina due to trichomonas, a parasitic flagellate protozoan organism or monilia, a type of fungi now known as candida). It is also used for surgical scrubbing and disinfection of instruments and endoscope. Povidone-iodine solution is generally used for disinfection of skin, mouth and throat. It is used as a solution, scrub solution, mouth wash, cream, ointment, vaginal pessary and also as an aerosol spray. Its another advantage is that it is easily washable from the skin.

Proprietory Preparations of Povidone-Iodine

    (a) PIODIN -1% mouth wash, 10% solution and 10% cream.

    (b) BETADIN-5% solution, 7.5% scrub solution, 5% ointment and 200 mg vaginal pessary.

    (c) RANVIDONE AEROSOL-5% aerosol spray with freon as propellant.

5. BORIC ACID

Refer Chapter 2.

6. BORAX, $Na_2B_4O_7 . 10H_2O$

Preparation: It is prepared from the mineral colemanite. It is boiled with concentrated sodium carbonate solution.

$$Ca_2B_6O_{11} + 2Na_2CO_3 \longrightarrow 2CaCO_3 + Na_2B_4O_7 + 2NaBO_2$$
$$\text{Borax} \qquad \text{Sodium}$$
$$\text{metaborate}$$

The solution is filitered and concentrated. Borax crystals separate. If a current of carbon dioxide is passed through the mother liquor, the metaborate also is converted into borax.

$$4NaBO_2 + CO_2 \longrightarrow Na_2CO_3 + Na_2B_4O_7$$

Physical and Chemical Properties: Borax occurs as a white crystalline powder without odour. It has a sweet alkaline taste. It is efflorescent in warm, dry air. It is slightly soluble in cold water but fairly soluble in hot water. It is soluble in glycerin.

On heating, it swells to form a white opaque mass and the anhydrous mass on heating to a high temperature (740°C) forms borax glass. Fused borax glass combines with metallic oxides to form metaborates which are highly coloured. Thus the reaction of borax glass with cobalt oxide gives cobalt metaborate which has an intense blue colour.

An aqueous solution of borax is distinctly alkaline to litmus and to phenolphthalein. This is because borax is hydrolysed to boric acid and sodium hydroxide. In concentrated solution, the hydrolysis is only partial but in dilute solution the hydrolysis is complete.

$$Na_2B_4O_7 + 3H_2O \rightleftharpoons 2NaBO_2 + 2H_3BO_3$$
$$\text{Sodium}$$
$$\text{metaborate}$$
$$NaBO_2 + 2H_2O \rightleftharpoons NaOH + H_3BO_3$$

When borax is treated with any mineral acid, boric acid is formed.

$$Na_2B_4O_7 + H_2SO_4 + 5H_2O \longrightarrow Na_2SO_4 + 4H_3BO_3$$

Excepting alkali metal borates, all the other metallic borates such as the calcium or barium borate are insoluble in water. It is official in B.P.1988.

Official Tests for Identity

1. To a solution prepared by dissolving the sample in carbon dioxide free water are added concentrated sulphuric acid and methanol and ignited. It burns with a green bordered flame. This is due to the formation of methyl borate.

2. To an aqueous solution is added phenolphthalein solution. A red colour is produced and it disappears on the addition of glycerol. The red colour is due to the alkaline reaction of borax. However the boric acid formed is converted to a stronger monobasic acid by glycerol which neutralises the alkalinity. So the red colour disappears.

3. An aqueous solution gives the reactions of sodium (see Chapter 13).

Standard: Borax (which is also known as sodium borate and sodium tetraborate) contains not less than 99 per cent and not more than 103 per cent of $Na_2B_4O_7 .10H_2O$.

Storage Condition: Since it is efflorescent, store in well-closed containers.

Chemical Incompatibility: Borax, because of its alkaline reaction, is incompatible with acids and substances which are hydrolysed by alkali such as oils. It is also incompatible with sodium bicarbonate and glycerol and carbon dioxide is evolved. Borax is also incompatible with calcium and barium salts, forming insoluble calcium and barium borates. It is incompatible also with soluble zinc salts and either insoluble basic zinc borate or zinc hydroxide is precipitated.

Assay: An accurately weighed quantity is added to mannitol solution in water, already neutralised to phenolphthalein. It is titrated with M/1 sodium hydroxide till a faint permanent pink colour is formed.

In this titration borax is hydrolysed to boric acid and the boric acid is converted by mannitol to mannityl boric acid, which is a stronger monobasic acid. The acid is titrated with molar sodium hydroxide solution. Any acidity present in mannitol is previously neutralised with M/10 sodium hydroxide solution using phenolphthalein as indicator.

Medicinal and Pharmaceutical Uses:

Antiseptic. Borax is mainly used in the preparation of vanishing creams and similar cosmetics.

It is also used in borax bead test for chemicals, in making optical and borosilicate glass and in making hard glass, glazes and enamel. It is also used as a flux in soldering and welding.

7. SILVER NITRATE, $AgNO_3$

Preparation: Silver nitrate is prepared by disssolving metallic silver in hot slightly concentrated nitric acid.

$$Ag + 2HNO_3 \longrightarrow AgNO_3 + NO_2\uparrow + H_2O$$

The solution is filtered through glass wool and set aside in a dark dust-proof room to crystallize. It is recrystallized from water.

Physical and Chemical Properties

Silver nitrate occurs as colourless or white rhombic or tabular crystals without odour and with a bitter, caustic, metallic taste. It is very soluble in water and sparingly soluble in alcohol. It is not affected by light, when pure. But when it comes into contact with any organic matter such as skin, it is reduced to metallic silver which is grey or greyish black in colour and leaves a stain. The best way to remove this stain is to paint it with tincture of iodine or any iodine solution and remove the iodine with a solution of sodium thiosulphate. When it is heated at 209°C, it melts to a slight yellow liquid without decomposition. However, on further heating, it slowly decomposes with evolution of oxides of nitrogen leaving a residue of metallic silver. Aqueous solution of silver nitrate is neutral to litmus. Silver nitrate is photo sensitive (affected by light).

On heating it gives metallic silver and nitrogen dioxide.

$$2Ag\,NO_3 \longrightarrow 2Ag + 2NO_2 + O_2$$

With ammonia it forms a complex known as silver diammino nitrate. The solution is known as ammoniacal silver nitrate and it is prepared by adding strong ammonia solution to silver nitrate solution till the black precipitate formed is dissolved.

$$AgNO_3 + 2NH_3 \longrightarrow Ag(NH_3)_2NO_3$$
$$\text{Silver diammino nitrate}$$

Further it answers the chemical reactions of silver and of the nitrate ion. Silver nitrate is official in I.P.

Official Tests for Identity :

A solution in water gives the reactions of silver and of nitrates (see Chapter 13).

Non-official Tests for Identity:

This test is for the nitrate ion. A dilute solution is mixed with a drop of diphenylamine and the mixture is added on a layer of concentrated sulphuric acid in a test tube. A blue colour is formed at the junction of the two layers.

Standard: Silver nitrate contains not less than 99.5 per cent and not more than 100.5 per cent of $AgNO_3$.

Storage Condition: Since silver nitrate is affected by light, store in tightly closed, light resistant (amber glass) containers.

Chemical Incompatibility: Silver nitrate is always externally used. It is incompatible with halides, cyanides and thiocyanates.

Medicinal and Pharmaceutical Uses

Local anti-infective: It is used in the form of eye drops for instillation in the eyes of newborn babies to guard against *Ophthalmia neonatorum*. Toughened silver nitrate (Lunar Caustic) containing about 95 per cent of silver nitrate is used for removing warts etc.

Ammoniacal silver nitrate is used as a reagent in the laboratory. Silver nitrate, besides its use in volumetric analysis, is also used for preparing silver halides used in photography and in silvering of mirrors.

8. MILD SILVER PROTEIN

Mild silver protein is silver rendered colloidal by combination with protein.

Preparation: Silver or silver oxide is reduced and subsequently made soluble in excess of denatured protein. It is dried in vacuum.

Properties: Mild silver protein occurs as dark brown to almost black shining scales or granules. It is odourless and has a tendency to be hygroscopic. It is freely soluble in water but almost insoluble in alcohol. It is affected by light and therefore should be protected from light.

Mild silver protein does not contain any free silver ions. This is evident from the fact that no opalescence will be formed when the filtrate from an alcoholic solution of mild silver protein is treated with dilute hydrochloric acid. For more chemical properties, see official tests for identity below. It is official in I.P.1966.

Official Tests for Identity.

1. A small quantity is heated till it is charred. It is completely incinerated and nitric acid is added to dissolve the greyish-white residue. The solution, after neutralisation, gives the reactions of silver (see Chapter 13).

2. Ferric chloride solution is added to a solution of the sample. The dark colour is discharged and the solution becomes opalescent on standing.

   Ferric chloride oxidises mild silver protein and the silver chloride formed gives the opalescence. Also the ferric and ferrous ions react with protein present to form an insoluble precipitate.

81

3. Mercuric chloride solution is added to a solution of mild silver protein. No white precipitate is produced and the liquid is not decolourised.

This test distinguishes mild silver protein from strong silver protein which precipitates the protein and gives a clear colourless supernatant liquid.

Standard: It contains not less than 19 per cent and not more than 23 per cent of Ag.

Storage Condition: As it is affected by light, mild silver protein should be stored in a well-closed container, protected from light in amber-glass containers.

Medicinal and Pharmaceutical Uses

Local anti-infective: It should be freshly prepared and dispensed. It is practically non-irritant and may be applied to tender mucous membranes. Used as a mild antiseptic in the eye, ear, nose and throat.

9. MERCURY, Hg

Mercury is known as quick silver and its symbol Hg comes from the Graeco-Latin word Hydrargyrum meaning liquid silver. It occurs as cinnabar, HgS and also in the free state in small globules in rocks and as silver and gold amalgam.

Preparation: Mercury is prepared by roasting cinnabar in a current of air in a shaft furnace or revolving furnace and the mercury vapour is condensed in brick lined chambers.

$$HgS + O_2 \longrightarrow Hg + SO_2$$

The mercury is filtered through chamois leather to remove dirt and dust and shaken with dilute nitric acid to remove metallic impurities like tin, lead, copper, zinc, silver etc.

Physical and Chemical Properties

Mercury is a bright, shining, silvery-white, heavy liquid which is easily divisible into small globules. It is extremely mobile and readily divisible into small globules. It readily volatilises on heating. It solidifies at $-39\ °C$ to a white, malleable, ductile solid and boils at

357°C. It has a specific gravity of 13.5. It expands rapidly and uniformly when heated and because of this nature it is widely used in making themometers, barometers etc. It is practically insoluble in water and alcohol. It is readily and completely soluble in concentrated sulphuric acid. Dilute and concentrated hydrochloric acid does not react with it.

Mercury forms two series of salts, the mercurous, derived from Hg_2O (mercurous oxide) and the mercuric, derived from HgO (mercuric oxide). They are both derived from ^+Hg — Hg^+ and Hg^+ ions respectively. Mercury usually tarnishes in air because of the metallic impurities present in it forming mercuric sulphide. At higher temperatures mercuric oxide is formed.

$$2Hg + O_2 \longrightarrow 2HgO$$

Hot concentrated sulphuric acid reacts with mercury to give either mercurous sulphate or mercuric sulphate depending upon the concentration of sulphuric acid and sulphur dioxide.

$$2Hg + 2H_2SO_4 \longrightarrow Hg_2SO_4 + SO_2\downarrow + 2H_2O$$
$$\text{Mercurous}$$
$$\text{sulphate}$$

$$Hg + 2H_2SO_4(\text{excess}) \longrightarrow HgSO_4 + SO_2\downarrow + 2H_2O$$
$$\text{Mercuric}$$
$$\text{sulphate}$$

Mercury forms amalgams with many metals such as sodium, silver, gold, tin, lead, copper, bismuth, cadmium, magnesium etc. Mercury is official in I.P.1966.

Official Tests for Identity

Refer Chapter 13 for reactions answered by mercurous and mercuric salts.

Standard: Mercury contains not less than 99.5 per cent of Hg.

Storage Condition: Store mercury in a strong well-closed container.

Medicinal and Pharmaceutical Uses: Topical anti-infective.

Previously mercury was used in the form of an ointment as a parasiticide and fungicide. Now it has been largely replaced by its compounds such as yellow mercuric oxide and ammoniated mercury.

Its other uses include its use in making thermometers, manometers, barometers etc., its use in preparing amalgams of metals, especially in the extraction of gold and silver and its use in mercury vapour lamps.

10. YELLOW MERCURIC OXIDE, HgO

Preparation: A concentrated solution of mercuric chloride is poured slowly with stirring into a dilute solution of sodium hydroxide. The mixture is allowed to stand for one hour at room temperature for complete reaction and also to allow the precipitate to settle. The supernatant liquid is decanted and the precipitate washed to remove alkali and chloride. It is then allowed to dry at room temperature. In the reaction between mercuric chloride and sodium hydroxide, the mercuric hydroxide first formed decomposes to give mercuric oxide.

$$HgCl_2 + 2NaOH \longrightarrow 2NaCl + Hg(OH)_2$$
$$\text{Mercuric hydroxide}$$

$$Hg(OH)_2 \longrightarrow HgO + H_2O$$
$$\text{Yellow}$$
$$\text{mercuric oxide}$$

Physical and Chemical Properties: This is a yellow to orange yellow, heavy, amorphous power. It is odourless and stable in air. It is converted into the red form by heating and remains red upon cooling. Exposure to light also gives the red form. It is practically insoluble in water and alcohol. It is readily soluble in dilute hydrochloric acid and in dilute nitric acid forming colourless solutions. The variation in colour between the red and yellow forms is due to difference in the size of the particles.

Mercuric oxide reacts with oleic acid to form mercury oleate, a salt of an organic acid. On strong heating it decomposes into oxygen and metallic mercury.

$$2HgO \longrightarrow 2Hg + O_2$$

As already stated it dissolves in dilute hydrochloric acid.

$$HgO + HCl \longrightarrow HgCl_2 + H_2O$$

It is official in I.P.1966.

Official Tests for Identity

1. When gently heated, it becomes red. When strongly heated, it decomposes into oxygen and mercury.

2. A solution in acid gives the reactions characteristic of mercuric salts (refer Chapter 13).

Standard: contains not less than 99.5 per cent of HgO, calculated with reference to the substance dried at 105°C for one hour.

Storage Condition: Store in a well-closed container, protected from light.

Assay: An accurately weighed quantity is dissolved in dilute nitric acid. The solution is titrated with N/10 ammonium thiocyanate using ferric ammonium sulphate as indicator.

In this assay, the mercuric oxide is converted into mercuric nitrate which is then titrated against ammonium thiocyanate.

$$HgO + 2HNO_3 \longrightarrow Hg(NO_3)_2 + H_2O$$

Mercuric
nitrate

$$2NH_4SCN + Hg(NO_3)_2 \longrightarrow Hg(SCN)_2 + NH_4NO_3$$

Ammonium   Mercuric
thiocyanate   thiocyanate

Medicinal and Pharmaceutical Use

Local anti-bacterial (ophthalmic). Because of a mild antiseptic action, it is used in ophthalmology for treating a number of inflammatory eye conditions.

11. AMMONIATED MERCURY, NH₂HgCl

Preparation: A cold solution of mercuric chloride is poured slowly with constant agitation into cold ammonia. The precipitate is washed with very dilute ammonia solution and dried in the dark below 30°C Washing is necessary to remove ammonium chloride but prolonged washing will give rise to a yellowish basic compound.

$$HgCl_2 + 2NH_3 \longrightarrow NH_2HgCl + NH_4Cl$$
Ammoniated
mercury

Physical and Chemical Properties: Ammoniated Mercury is a white amorphous powder which is odourless, it is stable in air but becomes dark on exposure to light. It has a styptic metallic taste. It is practically insoluble in water, alcohol and solvent ether. It is readily soluble in warm hydrochloric, nitric and acetic acids. It is gradually decomposed by prolonged washing with water, a yellow basic salt being produced.

It is decomposed by boiling alkalis completely.

$$NH_2HgCl + NaOH \longrightarrow NH_3 + HgO + NaCl$$

Ammoniated mercury reacts with potassium iodide in the presence of water as below:

$$NH_2HgCl + 2KI + H_2O \longrightarrow HgI_2 + NH_3 + KOH + KCl$$
Mercuric iodide

$$HgI_2 + 2KI \longrightarrow K_2HgI_4$$
Potassium mercuric iodide

It is official in I.P.'66.

Official Tests for Identity

1. Volatilises on being strongly heated without any fusion taking place.

2. Heat with sodium hydroxide solution. Yellow mercuric oxide is produced and ammonia is evolved.

3. A solution in acetic acid gives the reactions characteristic of mercuric salts, and of chlorides (refer Chapter 13).

Non-official Tests for Identity

1. The substance dissolves in sodium thiosulphate solution evolving ammonia.

2. Dissolve the sample in nitric acid and add potassium iodide solution. A red precipitate (mercuric iodide) is formed. It dissolves on adding excess of potassium iodide solution (refer assay).

Standard: Contains not less than 98 per cent of NH_2HgCl.

Storage Condition: Since it darkens on exposure to light, store ammoniated mercury in a well-closed container, protected from light.

Chemical Incompatibility: Ammoniated mercury is incompatible with alkalis and potassium iodide.

Assay: To the accurately weighed sample, water is added and also excess of potassium iodide. The mixture is shaken until solution is complete.

$$NH_2HgCl + 2KI + H_2O \longrightarrow HgI_2 + NH_3 + KOH + KCl$$

$$HgI_2 + 2KI \longrightarrow K_2HgI_4$$

The liberated ammonia and potassium hydroxide are titrated against N/10 hydrochloric acid, using methyl orange as indicator.

Medicinal and Pharmaceutical Use: Anti-infective.

C. SULPHUR AND ITS COMPOUNDS

Sulphur and its compounds are used as topical agents to treat scabies (precipitated sulphur and sublimed sulphur) and dandruff (selenium sulphide).

1. SUBLIMED SULPHUR, S.

Preparation: Sublimed sulphur or flowers of sulphur is prepared by heating sulphur in iron retorts and the vapour is allowed to go into large concrete chambers. The vapour becomes solid and falls to the ground as powder and also as friable masses. This is passed through sieves.

Physical and Chemical Properties. Sublimed sulphur is a fine yellow slightly gritty powder with a faint odour and without any taste. It burns with a blue flame forming sulphur dioxide. Under the microscope, sublimed sulphur appears as almost opaque rounded amorphous particles or aggregates, sometimes associated with semi-crystalline masses. It is almost insoluble in water and in alcohol. It is incompletely soluble in carbon disulphide. The I.P.1966 requires that not less than 20% of sublimed sulphur shall be insoluble in carbon disulphide. This is to prevent the possiblity of cheaper powdered sulphur (which is completely soluble in carbon disulphide) being used as an adulterant in sublimed sulphur.

Sulphur is a very active element and reacts with most metals and non-metals to form sulphides.

$$2Cu + S \longrightarrow Cu_2S$$

When sulphur burns in air, it forms suffocating fumes of sulphur dioxide.

$$S + O_2 \longrightarrow SO_2$$

Sulphur reacts with sulphites to give thiosulphates.

$$Na_2SO_3 + S \longrightarrow Na_2S_2O_3$$

When sulphur is boiled with calcium hydroxide solution, it forms a mixture of calcium polysulphide and calcium thiosulphate.

$$3Ca(OH)_2 + 6S \longrightarrow 2CaS_2 + CaS_2O_3 + 3H_2O$$
$$\text{Calcium} \quad \text{Calcium}$$
$$\text{polysulphide} \quad \text{thiosulphate}$$

The filtrate may be treated with enough hydrochloric acid to reprecipitate sulphur (refer preparation of precipitated sulphur).

$$2CaS_2 + CaS_2O_3 + 6HCl \longrightarrow 3CaCl_2 + 6S\downarrow + 3H_2O$$

It is official in I.P.1966.

Official Tests for Identity

A small quantity is heated. It melts at about 115°C to a yellow mobile liquid which becomes dark and viscid on further heating at about 160°C.

Storage Condition. Store in a well-closed container.

Medicinal and Pharmaceutical Uses. Used mainly as a **scabicide**. Sulphur ointment is prepared by using sublimed sulphur. The angular particles in sublimed sulphur open up the burrows of the skin sheltering the parasites which cause the scabies. Sulphur also acts as a mild antiseptic and parasiticide when rubbed into the skin.

2. PRECIPITATED SULPHUR, S.

Preparation

1. When a solution of a thiosulphate is acidified with a dilute mineral acid, thiosulphuric acid is formed. This is unstable and decomposes to form precipitated sulphur.

$$Na_2S_2O_3 + 2HCl \longrightarrow H_2S_2O_3 + 2NaCl$$
$$\text{Thiosulphuric}$$
$$\text{acid}$$

$$H_2S_2O_3 \longrightarrow S\downarrow + SO_2\uparrow + H_2O$$

2. Since thiosulphates are expensive, the following method is usually used for preparing precipitated sulphur. Slaked lime [$Ca(OH)_2$] is mixed with sublimed sulphur and water and it is boiled for one hour with occasional shaking. The liquid is filtered and the filtrate contains a mixture of thiosulphates and polysulphides. This is treated with enough hydrochloric acid to make the supernatant liquid slightly alkaline. The precipitated sulphur is filtered, washed on the filter to remove calcium and dried.

$$3Ca(OH)_2 + 6S \longrightarrow 2CaS_2 + CaS_2O_3 + 3H_2O$$

$$2CaS_2 + CaS_2O_3 + 6HCl \longrightarrow 3CaCl_2 + 6S\downarrow + 3H_2O$$

Physical and Chemical Properties. It is a pale greenish yellow to greyish yellow, soft powder. It should be free from grittiness. It is odourless and tasteless. It is completely soluble in carbon disulphide but almost insoluble in water and alcohol (90%).

The chemical properties of precipitated sulphur are the same as for sublimed sulphur. Precipitated sulphur is official in I.P.'66.

Official Test for Identity and Storage Condition: Same as for sublimed sulphur.

Medicinal Use: As a **scabicide**.

3. SELENIUM SULPHIDE, SeS_2

Properties: A bright orange to reddish brown powder with an odour faintly resembling that of hydrogen sulphide. It is official in B.P.1988.

89

Official Tests for Identity

1. A small quantity is boiled with concentrated nitric acid, diluted with water and filtered. To the filtrate is added urea. It is boiled and cooled. Potassium iodide solution is added. A yellow to orange colour, which darkens rapidly on standing, is produced.

2. The coloured solution obtained in (1) above is allowed to stand for 10 minutes and filtered through kieselguhr. The filtrate gives the reactions of sulphates.

Standard: Selenium sulphide contains not less than 52 per cent and not more than 55 per cent of Se.

Storage Condition: Store in a well-closed container.

Medicinal Use: Used in the treatment of dandruff and seborrhoeic dermatitis of the scalp.

It is available as Selsun Cream (0.5%) and Selsun Suspension (a 2.5% shampoo).

In these preparations, selenium sulphide is non-irritant and is not absorbed significantly.

D. ASTRINGENTS

An astringent, as mentioned earlier, hardens and protects the skin by precipitating proteins. The following two substances are important astringents.

1. ALUM (POTASH SLUM, ALUMINIUM POTASSIUM SULPHATE), $KAI (SO_4)_2, 12H_2O$

Alum is either potash alum or ammonia alum. An alum is a double salt of a trivalent element and an univalent element with 12 molecules of water of hydration. The trivalent elements are ususally iron, aluminium, chromium, manganese etc.and the univalent elements may be sodium, potassium, or ammonium. Alum of the pharmacopeia (official in I.P.1966 and B.P.1988) is potash alum i.e. a double salt of aluminium sulphate and potassium sulphate with 12 molecules of water of hydration.

Preparation: Potash alum is prepared by adding a hot, concentrated solution of potassium sulphate to a hot solution of an equivalent quantity of aluminium sulphate. The solution is cooled and the alum crystallizes out. By crystallizing slowly it is possible to get large, regular, octahedral crystals.

$$Al_2(SO_4)_3.18\ H_2O + K_2SO_4 \longrightarrow 2KAl(SO_4)_2.12H_2O + 6H_2O$$
$$\text{Potash alum}$$

Physical and Chemical Properties

Alum occurs as large, octahedral, colourless crystals or in small crystals or as a white powder. It is without odour and has a sweetish, strongly astringent taste. Alum is soluble in cold water but more soluble in hot water. Alum is transparent but it is sometimes opaque on the surface due to traces of basic salt being formed. When basic salt is present, alum will not give a clear solution. When alum is heated, it melts at 92°C and loses all the water of hydration at 200°C leaving a white residue known as burnt alum containing anhydrous aluminum and potassium sulphates.

Official Tests for Identity

1. A solution in water gives the reactions characteristic of aluminium and sulphates (see chapter 13).

2. A small quantity of a solution in water is treated with sodium bicarbonate and filtered. The filtrate gives the reactions of potassium (see chapter 13).

Standard: Alum contains not less than 99 per cent and not more than 100.5 per cent of KAl $(SO_4)_2$, $12H_2O$.

Storage Conditon: Alum should be stored in a well - closed container.

Chemical Incompatibility: Alum is incompatible with proteins, precipitating them. This is utilised in preparing certain biological preparations such as alum precipitated tetanus toxoid and alum precipitated diphtheria toxoid.

Medicinal and Pharmaceutical Uses

Astringent. Alum precipitates proteins and protects and hardens the skin. It is used to prepare styptic pencil used for stopping the bleeding in small cuts.

2. ZINC SULPHATE, ZnSO$_4$. 7H$_2$O

Preparation: It is prepared by boiling a slight excess of metallic zinc with dilute sulphuric acid.

$$Zn + H_2SO_4 \longrightarrow ZnSO_4 + H_2$$

The liquid is filtered and evaporated to crystallization.

Properties: Zinc sulphate occurs as colourless, transparent crystals, or as a crystalline powder. It is odourless and has an astringent, metallic taste. It is efflorescent in dry air. It is easily soluble in water, insoluble in alcohol and soluble in glycerin. It combines with potassium and ammonium sulphates to form double salts, M$_2$SO$_4$. ZnSO$_4$. 6H$_2$O.

Aqueous solution of zinc sulphate is slightly acidic.

It is official in I.P.

Official Tests for Identity: Gives the reactions characteristic of zinc, and of sulphates (refer Chapter 13).

Standard: Contains the equivalent of not less than 99.0 per cent and not more than 108 per cent of the hydrated salt, ZnSO$_4$.7H$_2$O.

Storage condition: Since it is efflorescent, store in a well-closed contianer.

Assay: An accuratly weighed quantity is dissolved in water and strong ammonia-ammonium chloride buffer is added. It is titrated against M/20 disodium ethylenediaminetetraacetate using eriochrome black T as indicator.

This is a complexometric assay like the assay of magnesium sulphate. The end point is the appearance of deep blue colour.

Medicinal Use: Emetic (induces vomiting) and astringent.

CHAPTER 6

CONSUMER DENTAL PRODUCTS

Consumer dental products include dentifrices (tooth powders, tooth pastes and liquid dentifrices), mouth washes and rinses, toothache drops, denture adhesives and denture cleaners. The compounds considered below may be used for the preparation of one or more of the above classes of dental products and some of them like sodium fluoride are also used for toughening the tooth enamel against dental caries.

1. SODIUM FLUORIDE, NaF

Preparation: Sodium fluoride is made by the reaction of sodium carbonate with hydrofluoric acid.

$$2HF + Na_2CO_3 \longrightarrow 2NaF + H_2O + CO_2\uparrow$$

Physical and Chemical Properties

Sodium fluoride occurs as colourless crystals or as a white powder. It is slightly soluble in water but practically insoluble in alcohol. Aqueous solutions of sodium fluoride may corrode glass bottles. It should not be stored for more than six months.

Poisonous hydrofluoric acid is produced when sodium flouride solution is acidified. This acid attacks glass. Aqueous solution of sodium fluoride is alkaline in reaction. Sodium flouride forms stable complexes with ferric iron and its assay method is based on this reaction. It is official in B.P.1988.

Official Tests for Identity

1. A solution of the sample in carbon dioxide–free water is treated with calcium chloride solution. A gelatinous white precipitate is produced. It dissolves on adding ferric chloride solution.

2. To a small quantity of the sample is added alizarin red solution and zirconyl nitrate solution. A red lake is produced. It soon changes to yellow.

93

3. Gives the reactions characteristic of sodium (see Chapter 13).

Standard: Sodium fluoride contains not less than 98.5 per cent and not more than 100.5 per cent of NaF, calculated with reference to the dried substance.

Storage Condition: Sodium flouride should be stored only in pyrex glass bottles. It should not be stored for more than six months.

Medicinal and Pharmaceutical Uses

Used for retarding or preventing dental caries and tooth decay. About 1 to 1.5 p.p.m. (parts per million) of sodium fluoride may be included in tooth pastes for this purpose for toughening the tooth enamel.

2. STANNOUS FLUORIDE, SnF_2

It can be prepared by dissolving stannous hydroxide in hydrofluoric acid and evaporating the solution in the absence of air. It is a white crystalline substance. It is said to be better than sodium fluoride in preventing dental caries.

3. CALCIUM CARBONATE, $CaCO_3$

See under Antacids - Chapter 4.

Precipitated calcium carbonate is very useful as the standard abrasive ingredient in tooth powders and tooth pastes.

4. SODIUM METAPHOSPHATE, $NaPO_3$

Sodium metaphosphate is prepared by heating primary sodium phosphate (sodium dihydrogen phosphate)

$$NaH_2PO_4 \longrightarrow NaPO_3 + H_2O$$

It is a transparent, glassy solid. Its aqueous solution gives a white gelatinous precipitate with magnesia mixture or cobalt nitrate solution. It also gives a white precipitate with barium chloride in hydrochloric acid.

5. DIBASIC CALCIUM PHOSPHATE, CaHPO$_4$ or CaHPO$_4$, 2H$_2$O

Dibasic calcium phosphate or dicalcium phosphate is the anhydrous substance (CaHPO$_4$) or a crystalline salt containing two molecules of water of hydration (CaHPO$_4$, 2H$_2$O).

Preparation: It is prepared by the interaction of secondary sodium phosphate (disodium hydrogen phosphate) and calcium chloride in a neutral solution.

$$Na_2 HPO_4 + CaCl_2 \longrightarrow Ca HPO_4\downarrow + 2NaCl$$

Properties : It is a white powder which is odourless and tasteless. It is stable in air. It is practically insoluble in water and alcohol but soluble in dilute nitric acid. It is official in I.P.

Official Tests for Identity

1. A solution in warm dilute hydrochloric acid gives the reactions of calcium (see Chapter 13).

2. A solution in warm, dilute nitric acid gives the reactions of phosphates (see chapter 13)

Standard: Dibasic calcium phosphate contains not less than 30.9 per cent and not more than 31.7 per cent of Ca, calculated with reference to the ignited substance.

Storage Condition: Since it is stable in air, store in well closed containers.

Chemical Incompatibility

It is incompatible with alkalis and bases such as sodium bicarbonate, evolving carbon dioxide.

Medicinal and Pharmaceutical Uses

Dibasic calcium phosphate may be used partially to replace precipitated calcium carbonate in formulas for tooth powders and tooth pastes. It is also used to treat calcium and phosphorous deficiency states.

6. ZINC CHLORIDE, ZnCl$_2$

Preparation: Zinc metal or zinc oxide or zinc carbonate is treated with hydrochloric acid to form the zinc chloride.

$$ZnO + 2HCl \longrightarrow ZnCl_2 + H_2O$$

Physical and Chemical Properties: Zinc chloride occurs as white or nearly white, crystalline powder or granules. It is also available as fused sticks or pencils. It is odourless and very deliquescent. It is very soluble in water and freely soluble in alcohol. The solutions are slightly turbid due to the formation of the carbonate. They become clear on the addition of dilute hydrochloric acid. At 290°C zinc chloride fuses to a clear liquid. At about 750°C a part of it is volatilized. The rest is decomposed and leaves a residue of zinc oxide.

Aqueous solution of zinc chloride is acid to litmus due to hydrolysis. Zinc chloride forms auto-complex halides. Auto-complex halides are salts in which the same metal is attached to both anion and cation.

$$2ZnCl_2 \rightleftharpoons Zn(ZnCl_4)$$

Official Tests for Identity

1. A solution in very dilute hydrochloric acid gives the reactions of zinc (see Chapter 13).

2. A solution in very dilute nitric acid gives the reactions of chloride (see Chapter 13).

Standard: Zinc chloride contains not less than 95 per cent and not more than 100.5 per cent of ZnCl$_2$.

Storage Condition: Since it is very deliquescent, store in tightly closed containers.

Medicinal and Pharmaceutical Uses: Zinc chloride is used in mouth washes for its **antiseptic and astringent** properties. It is also used for preparing zinc insulins.

7. STRONTIUM CHLORIDE, SrCl$_2$.6H$_2$O

Preparation: Strontium chloride is prepared by reacting hydrochloric acid with the oxide, hydroxide or carbonate of strontium.

$$SrO + 2HCl \longrightarrow SrCl_2 + H_2O$$
$$Sr(OH)_2 + 2HCl \longrightarrow SrCl_2 + 2H_2O$$
$$SrCO_3 + 2HCl \longrightarrow SrCl_2 + H_2O + CO_2\uparrow$$

The solution is then filtered, concentrated and allowed to crystallize.

Properties: It consists of colourless, odourless crystals or white granules. It effloresces in dry air and is readily soluble in water and alcohol.

Storage Condition: Since it effloresces in dry air, store in well-closed containers.

Medicinal or Pharmaceutical Use: Desensitizer

It is used to reduce sensitivity of teeth to heat and cold. When there is tooth ache or tooth decay, teeth are more sensitive to heat or cold. In this connection, strontium chloride acts like zinc chloride. It is possible that they may act like local anesthetics to prevent the perception of heat and cold by the teeth.

CHAPTER 7

INHALANTS AND RESPIRATORY STIMULANTS

A. INHALANTS

The inhalants dealt with in this chapter are medical gases, that is, oxygen, carbon dioxide and nitrous oxide. They are filled into steel cylinders which are subject to Indian and International standards. Thus the cylinders should be able to withstand a pressure of 3000 lb per sq inch (at least 2000 lb per sq inch) and follow a colour code prescribed for this purpose.

1. OXYGEN, O_2

Oxygen is essential to animal and human life. It constitutes about 21 per cent of the atmosphere and 50 per cent of the terrestrial matter. Plants take up carbon dioxide and liberate oxygen during photosynthesis.

Preparation: Oxygen is usually prepared by the fractional distillation of liquid air. It is also prepared by the electrolysis of water.Since water is a non-conductor of electricity, sodium hydroxide solution is used, Iron electrodes are used and the oxygen and hydrogen produced are collected separately.

Physical and Chemical Properties

Oxygen is a colourless, tasteless and odourless gas. It is slightly heavier than air. It can be liquefied at $-118.8°C$. It is sparingly soluble in water (1 in 32) but is freely soluble in alcohol (1 in 3.5). Oxygen stimulates a glowing splinter to burn brightly with a flame. Oxygen is one of the most active elements. At about 5000°C the molecular form of oxygen (O_2) dissociates into the atomic form (O) completely. The atomic form of oxygen is much more active than the molecular form. It is also formed during oxidation reactions such as those involving acidified potassium permangante. Oxygen combines with most metals directly. If a catalyst is present, the reaction is stimulated to a great extent.

$$S + O_2 \longrightarrow SO_2\uparrow$$

$$C + O_2 \longrightarrow CO_2\uparrow$$

$$4Fe + 3O_2 \xrightarrow{\Delta} 2Fe_2O_3$$

$$2Mg + O_2 \xrightarrow{\Delta} 2MgO$$

Magnesium ribbon burns in oxygen forming magnesium oxide. Oxidative changes are brought about by oxygen of the atmosphere in paints, oils and fats etc. This can be prevented by including antioxidants in the preparations. Oxygen is official in I.P.

Official Tests for Identity

1. Oxygen causes a glowing splinter to burn brightly.

2. Oxygen is absorbed when it is shaken with alkaline pyrogallol solution. The solution turns dark brown.

3. When oxygen is mixed with an equal volume of nitric oxide red fumes are produced (distinction from nitrous oxide).

Standard: Oxygen contains not less than 99 per cent v/v of O_2.

Storage Condition: Oxygen should be stored under compression in appropriate metal cylinders with prescribed safety regulations. Valves should not be lubricated with oil or grease. The shoulder of the metal cylinder should be painted white and the rest is painted black. The name of the gas should be on the label and also painted on the shoulder of the cylinder.

Medicinal and Pharmaceutical Uses

Medical Gas: Oxygen is essential for breathing. Whenever there is any respiratory difficulty, as in asthma or pneumonia, oxygen is administered. It is also used during surgery. It is administered along with helium or with carbon dioxide. Liquid oxygen is used for removing warts.

2. CARBON DIOXIDE, CO_2

Carbon dioxide is present in the atmosphere to the extent of about 0.03%. It is a product of combustion, respiration and fermentation reactions.

Preparation:

1. It may be prepared by heating alkali carbonates and bicarbonates.

$$2NaHCO_3 \longrightarrow Na_2CO_3 + CO_2\uparrow + H_2O$$

2. It may also be prepared by the action of acids on carbonates or bicarbonates.

$$Na_2CO_3 + H_2SO_4 \longrightarrow Na_2SO_4 + CO_2\uparrow + H_2O$$

Carbon dioxide is also formed from the products of combustion of coke, from fermentation and during the manufacture of lime by burning limestone in lime kilns.

Physical and Chemical Properties

Carbon dioxide is a colourless and odourless gas. It is freely soluble in water (1 in 1) and the aqueous solution, known as aerated water (soda) has a faintly acid taste. It is about one and a half times heavier than air. It can be easily liquefied under a pressure of about 50 to 60 atmospheres and this liquid becomes solid at $-57.7°C$. The so-called "dry ice" is solid carbon dioxide.

Carbon dioxide does not support combusion. A burning splinter is extinguished when it is introduced into a jar containing carbon dioxide. It dissolves in water to form carbonic acid which is, however, unstable.

$$CO_2 + H_2O \rightleftharpoons H_2CO_3$$

Carbonic acid, being a dibasic acid, forms both acid and normal salts.

$$NaOH + H_2CO_3 \longrightarrow NaHCO_3 + H_2O$$

$$NaHCO_3 + NaOH \longrightarrow Na_2CO_3 + H_2O$$

Carbonic acid reddens blue litmus. When carbon dioxide is passed into a solution of calcium hydroxide (lime water), the solution turns milky due to the formation of calcium carbonate. On passing more carbon dioxide, the liquid becomes clear due to the formation of calcium bicarbonate. If this solution is heated, carbon dioxide is liberated and the solution again turns milky due to the reprecipitation of calcium carbonate.

$$Ca(OH)_2 + CO_2 \longrightarrow CaCO_3 + H_2O$$
$$CaCO_3 + H_2O + CO_2 \longrightarrow Ca(HCO_3)_2$$
$$Ca(HCO_3)_2 \longrightarrow CaCO_3 + H_2O + CO_2\uparrow$$

When passed through reduced coke, carbon dioxide is reduced to carbon monoxide.

$$CO_2 + C \longrightarrow 2CO$$

It is official in B.P. 1988.

Official Tests for Identity

1. Carbon dioxide extinguishes a burning splinter.

2. When the gas is passed through a solution of barium hydroxide, a white precipitate (barium carbonate) is produced. It dissolves with effervescence on the addition of dilute acetic acid.

Standard: Carbon dioxide contains not less than 99 percent v/v of CO_2.

Storage Condition: Carbon dioxide should be kept liquefied under pressure in approved metal cylinders. The metal cylinder should be painted grey and carry a label stating 'carbon dioxide'. In addition 'Carbon dioxide' or the symbol 'CO_2' should be stencilled in paint on the shoulder of the cylinder.

Medicinal and Pharmaceutical Uses

Medical Gas: Carbon dioxide (5%) is used along with oxygen to stimulate respiration when it is depressed in poisoning by carbon monoxide and by drugs such as morphine. It is used for manufacturing some chemicals such as sodium bicarbonate, sodium carbonate etc. Soda water (water containing carbon dioxide under pressure) acts as a carminative and promotes absorption in the stomach.

3. NITROUS OXIDE, N_2O

Preparation: Nitrous oxide is prepared by heating ammonium nitrate. Since ammonium nitrate may explode when strongly heated, a mixture of sodium nitrate and ammonium sulphate may be used.

$$NH_4NO_3 \longrightarrow N_2O\uparrow + 2H_2O$$

$$2NaNO_3 + (NH_4)_2SO_4 \longrightarrow 2N_2O\uparrow + 4H_2O + Na_2SO_4$$

The gas is collected over hot water. It may be purified by passing through ferrous sulphate solution (to remove higher oxides of nitrogen), caustic soda solution (to remove nitric acid) and concentrated sulphuric acid (to remove water vapour).

Physical and Chemical Properties

Nitrous oxide is a colourless, odourless and tasteless gas. It is about one and a half times heavier than air. It is soluble in water and freely soluble in alcohol. It is liquefied to a thin, mobile colourless liquid which boils at $-89.5°C$. The liquid freezes to a white solid at $-102.4°C$. It produces exhilarating effects or hysterical laughter when inhaled. Hence it is known as 'laughing gas'.

On heating it decomposes into nitrogen and oxygen.

$$2N_2O \longrightarrow 2N_2 + O_2$$

It does not support combustion. However since it is readily decomposed, the oxygen released from it supports the combusion of a burning splinter, burning phosphorus and burning sulphur.

$$C + 2N_2O \longrightarrow CO_2 + 2N_2$$

$$S + 2N_2O \longrightarrow SO_2 + 2N_2$$

Nitrous oxide is reduced to nitrogen when it is passed over hot copper.

$$Cu + N_2O \longrightarrow CuO + N_2$$

It is official in I.P.

Official Tests for Identity

1. A glowing wood splinter bursts into flames when introduced into the gas.

2. The gas is not absorbed by alkaline pyrogallol solution.

Standard: Nitrous oxide contains not less than 95 per cent v/v of N_2O in the gaseous phase.

Storage Condition: Nitrous oxide is stored under compression in metal cylinders of the type conforming to the appropriate safety regulations and at a temperature not exceeding 37°C. The cylinder is painted blue and carries a label with the name of the gas or N_2O which is also painted on the shoulder of the cylinder.

Medicinal and Pharmaceutical Uses

Medical Gas. General anaesthetic (inhalation) and analgesic

It is used to carry out minor operations such as tooth extractions and removal of boils and abscesses. It is also used for calming excited mental patients. It is used in a concentration of 60 - 80% along with oxygen in a concentration of 20 - 40%. Since it does not combine with haemoglobin, nitrous oxide is also used to measure the cerebral and coronary blood flow.

B. RESPIRATORY STIMULANT

Reflex stimulation of the central nervous system is brought about by subjecting the patient to inhalation of substances like ammonium carbonate which gives off ammonia in conditions of syncope or fainting. In other words a person who has fainted is revived by keeping ammonium carbonate or any other volatile ammonium salt near his nose. These substances are also known as smelling salts.

AMMONIUM CARBONATE, NH_4HCO_3, NH_4COONH_2

Ammonium carbonate is also known as *ammonium sesquicarbonate and sal volatile*. It is a variable mixture of ammonium bicarbonate (NH_4HCO_3)and ammonium carbamate (NH_4COONH_2). It contains not less than 30 per cent of ammonia.

Preparation: Ammonium carbonate may be prepared by subliming a mixture of ammonium sulphate or ammonium chloride with chalk (calcium carbonate) in iron retorts and condensing the vapour in chambers lined with lead. The ammonia produced along with the ammonium carbonate is recovered by passing into sulphuric acid.

$$2(NH_4)_2SO_4 + 2CaCO_3 \longrightarrow NH_4HCO_3 . NH_4COONH_2$$
$$+ NH_3 + H_2O + 2CaSO_4$$

Physical and Chemical Properties

Ammonium carbonate consists of hard, traslucent (semi-transparent), crystalline masses with a strong ammoniacal odour. It has a pungent and ammoniacal taste. It is soluble in water and partly soluble in alcohol. A residue of ammonium bicarbonate is found at the bottom of the alcoholic solution confirming the partial solubility. Aqueous solutions of the salt are alkaline.

When it is exposed to air, it partially dissociates and volatilises getting converted into porous opaque lumps or into a white powder. The residue is mainly ammonium bicarbonate. Ammonia and carbon dioxide are given off.

$$NH_4HCO_3 .NH_4COONH_2 \longrightarrow 2NH_3\uparrow + CO_2\uparrow + NH_4HCO_3$$

The same result is produced by dissolving it in hot water.

When it is treated with dilute ammonia, it is readily converted to the normal carbonate $(NH_4)_2CO_3$.

$$NH_4HCO_3 .NH_4COONH_2 + NH_4OH \longrightarrow 2(NH_4)_2CO_3$$

It is decomposed by the addition of any mineral acid. The acid may be added to the dry salt or to a solution of the salt in water.

$$NH_4HCO_3. NH_4 COONH_2 + 3HCl \longrightarrow 3NH_4Cl + H_2O + 2CO_2\uparrow$$

Ammonium carbonate is not official in B.P. or I.P.

Tests for Identity

1. When a little of the salt is heated, it is volatilised and no charring takes place. When tested with moist litmus paper, the vapour is strongly alkaline.

2. When a dilute mineral acid is added to an aqueous solution of the salt, effervescence is produced.

Storage Condition: Since it is volatile, store in a tightly closed container.

Chemical Incompatibility: It is incompatible with acids or acidic substances. Carbon dioxide is evolved. It is also incompatible with alkaloidal salts.

Medicinal and Pharmaceutical Uses: Respiratory Stimulant

As already stated, it is used for the revival of the fainted patients by reflex stimulation of their central nervous system by inhalation. It is also used as an expectorant and antacid.

CHAPTER 8

EXPECTORANTS, EMETICS AND ANTIDOTES

A. EXPECTORANTS AND EMETICS

Expectorants are drugs which enhance the secretion of the sputum by the air passages so that it is easier to remove the phlegm through coughing. They are used in cough mixtures for this purpose. They act either by increasing the bronchial secretion or by making it less viscous (mucolytic agents). Drugs such as as ipecacuanha in small doses act as stimulant expectorants. They irritate the lining of the stomach which reflexly stimulates the production of sputum by the glands in the bronchial mucous membrane. If given in high doses, they act as emetics, that is they induce vomiting.

Potassium iodide stimulates the gastric mucosa and reflexly increases the bronchial secretions. Ammonium chloride acts like potassium iodide but is less potent. Antimony potassium tartrate also is used as an expectorant. But it has gone out of use as an emetic (a drug inducing vomiting) since better and safer drugs are now available for the purpose.

1. AMMONIUM CHLORIDE, NH_4Cl

Preparation: Ammonium chloride is made by reacting hydrochloric acid with ammonia. The solution is evaporated to dryness.

$$NH_3 + HCl \longrightarrow NH_4Cl$$

The product is purified by recrystallization or by sublimation.

Physical and Chemical Properties: Crude ammonium chloride or sal ammoniac consists of tough, crystalline masses. The pure substance is a white crystalline powder. It is odourless with a saline taste. It is freely soluble in water.

When heated, ammonium chloride volatilises. It is considered to decompose into ammonia and hydrochloric acid but the components reunite when cooled. This phenomenon can be seen when ammonium chloride is heated in a test tube. Ammonia and hydrochloric acid formed at the bottom due to the decomposition of ammonium chloride reunite at the top of the test tube to form a white deposit.

$$NH_4Cl \rightleftharpoons NH_3 + HCl$$

Due to this dissociation, ammonium chloride is used as a flux in soldering for removing the film of oxide from the surface of the metal. The HCl formed converts the metallic oxide into chloride which, being volatile, is driven off easily at the high temperature. Even though ammonium chloride solution is neutral when freshly prepared, it becomes slightly acid on standing due to hydrolysis.

It is official in I.P.

Official Tests for Identity

Gives the reactions characteristic of ammonium salts and of chlorides (refer Chapter 13).

Standard: Contains not less than 99.5 per cent of NH_4Cl calculated with reference to the substance dried over silica gel for four hours.

Storage Condition: Since ammonium chloride is slightly hygroscopic, it is stored in a well closed container.

Chemical Incompatibility: Due to the slightly acid reaction of the aqueous solution of ammonium chloride on standing, it is incompatible with basic substances.

Assay: I.P. 1985 gives the following method.

Formaldehyde, previously neutralised to phenolphthalein, is added to a solution of the substance. It fixes the ammonia in ammonium chloride as hexamine. The liberated hydrochloric acid is titrated against N/10 sodium hydroxide,using phenolphthalein as indicator.

A modified Volhard's method was used in I.P.'66. A solution of the substance, acidified with nitric acid, is shaken with a measured volume of N/10 silver nitrate, nitrobenzene being previously added. Nitrobenzene is added to coagulate the precipitate of silver chloride, so that it will not interfere with the titration later of excess of silver nitrate which is determined by titration with N/10 ammonium thiocyanate, using ferric ammonium sulphate as indicator.

$$AgNO_3 + NH_4Cl \longrightarrow AgCl + NH_4NO_3$$

$$AgNO_3 + NH_4SCN \longrightarrow AgSCN + NH_4NO_3$$

Ammonium   Silver
thiocyanate.   thiocyanate.

The following is the reaction taking place at the end point when red ferric thiocyanate is formed (by reaction of ammonium thiocyanate with the indicator ferric amminum sulphate).

$$Fe\,NH_4(SO_4)_2 + 3NH_4\,SCN \longrightarrow Fe(SCN)_3 + 2(NH_4)_2SO_4$$

Ferric ammonium   Ammonium   Ferric
sulphate   thiocyanate   thiocyante

Medicinal Use: Expectorant, diuretic and systemic acidifier

2. POTASSIUM IODIDE, KI

Preparation: Potassium iodide is prepared by adding a slight excess of iodine to a solution of potassium hydroxide to form a mixture of potassium iodide and iodate. The iodate is reduced completely to iodide by heating with charcoal.

$$6KOH + 3I_2 \longrightarrow 5KI + KIO_3 + 3H_2O$$

$$KIO_3 + 3C \longrightarrow KI + 3CO$$

Physical and Chemical Properties: Potassium iodide occurs as large, transparent and colourless or white and somewhat opaque cubes or as a white, granular powder. It is odourless and has a saline and slightly bitter taste. It is stable in dry air. It is very soluble in water (1 in 0.7) and soluble in alcohol (1 in 23). Aqueous solutions of potassium iodide take up iodine, when the iodine is dissolved in them and form KI_3 which is in equilibrium with dissolved iodine.

$$KI_3 \rightleftharpoons KI + I_2$$

Potassium iodide deliquesces slightly in moist air. It answers all the chemical reactions of the iodide ion (refer Chapter 13). It is official in I.P.

Official Tests for Identity: Gives the reactions characteristic of potassium and of iodides (refer Chapter 13).

Standard: Contains not less than 99.5 per ent of KI, calculated with reference to the substance dried to constant weight at 105°C.

Storage Condition: Since potassium iodide is slightly deliquescent, it is stored in a well closed container.

Chemical Incompatibility: Potassium iodide is incompatible with oxidizing agents such as ferric iron and potassium chlorate. It is oxidized to iodine which is liberated. Potassium iodide is also incompatible with some alkaliods like quinine. Quinine mixed with potassium iodide and dilute sulphuric acid undergoes 'herapathite reaction' and forms olive green scales of a substance known as 'herapathite'. However this reaction is slow and it takes more than three days for the herapathite to be formed.

Medicinal and Pharmaceutical Uses

Expectorant and as a source of iodine. This is also an ingredient in many laboratory reagents, such as Mayer's Reagent and Nessler's Reagent.

3. ANTIMONY POTASSIUM TARTRATE, KOOC-CHOH-CHOH -COO (SbO), $^1/_2$ H_2O

Preparation: It is prepared by mixing antimonious oxide and finely powdered potassium acid tartrate and making into a paste. It is set aside overnight. Then after adding water, it is boiled, filtered and the filtrate allowed to crystallize. The crystals are dried at room temperature.

$$Sb_2O_3 + 2 \quad \begin{array}{c} KOOC\text{---}CHOH \\ | \\ HOOC\text{---}CHOH \end{array}$$

Potassium acid tartrate

$\downarrow$

$$2 \quad \begin{array}{c} KOOC\text{-------}CHOH \\ | \\ (OSb)OOC\text{------}CHOH \end{array} \quad . \quad \tfrac{1}{2}H_2O$$

Antimony potassium tartrate

Physical and Chemical Properties

Antimony potassium tartrate consists of colourless, transparent crystals or occurs as a white granular powder. It is odourless and has a sweet taste. The crystals effloresce on exposure to air. It is soluble in water and insoluble in alcohol.

Its aqueous solution is only slightly acid but it is enough to turn the blue litmus paper red. It has the advantage over other antimony compounds that it does not deposit insoluble basic compounds on dilution or when it is boiled with water. It is a trivalent antimony compound and it is easily oxidised by iodine to the pentavalent state. This is the assay method for antimony potassium tartrate.

$$KOOC-CHOH-CHOH-COO(SbO) + I_2 + 2H_2O \longrightarrow$$

$$HSbO_3 + 2HI + KOOC - CHOH - CHOH - COOH$$

Metantimonic acid   Potassium acid tartrate

Antimony potassium tartrate was last official in B.P. 1953.

Official Tests for Identity: Gives the reactions characteristic of antimony and potassium. After removal of the antimony it gives the reactions of tartrates (see Chapter 13).

Storage Condition: Since it is efflorescent, store in a well closed container.

Chemical Incompatibility: Antimony potassium tartrate is a trivalent antimony compound which is incompatible with oxidising agents like iodine.

Medicinal and Pharmaceutical Use

Emetic. Also used as a depressant expectorant in small doses. It is also useful as an intravenous injection in the treatment of diseases like kala-azar and schistosomiasis.

B. ANTIDOTES

4. SODIUM NITRITE, NaNO3

Refer Chapter 3.

CHAPTER 9

MAJOR INTRA AND
EXTRA-CELLULAR ELECTROLYTES

Water forms the major part of the human body mass. Thus while the male contains about 60 per cent of water, the female contains about 51 per cent. This water is divided in the body into two major compartments–the extracellular fluid (ECF) and the intracellular fluid (ICF). The ECF is further subdivided into intravascular fluid (plasma) which is present inside the blood vessels and the extravascular fluid outside the blood vessels which comprises of interstitial fluid, lymph etc. Intracellular fluid is the fluid present within the cells. Almost all cell membranes are freely permeable to water, that is they allow the passage of water freely.

ELECTROLYTE BALANCE

The plasma (that is, the blood) is in equilibrium with the extracellular fluid outside the blood vessels known as the interstitial fluid. The endothelium (membrane) of the blood vessels acts as a semipermeable membrane and allows the passage of water and most of the solutes in the blood.

Electrolytes are inorganic salts present in solution as charged ions that is, cations (positively charged) and anions (negatively charged). They are present in blood and maintain the osmotic pressure of the blood. Because of this osmotic pressure there is no passage of water across the cell membrane. Therefore it is essential that the osmotic pressure be maintained at a particular level so that blood may flow within the blood vessels without being attracted via the cell membrane into the interstitial fluid (extravascular fluid).

Actually the cell membrane separates two fluids (blood and interstitial fluid) of different composition but which have equal osmotic pressure. The plasma contains a large quantity of sodium ions and a small quanity each of potassium, calcium and magnesium ions. The anions present include a good amount of chloride and bicarbonate and a small quantity of phosphate, organic anions and some amount of proteins. The table given below gives the actual quantity of the ions present in plasma in mEQ/litre.

Electrolytes Present in Plasma

Cations (mEq/l)		Anions (mEq/l)	
Sodium	135-145	Chloride	98-106
Potassium	3.5-5	Bicarbonate	24-28
Calcium	4.5-5.3	Phosphate	2-5
Magnesium	1.5-2.0	Organic anions	3-6
		Proteins	15-20

The volume of the extracellular fluid (ECF) including blood, its electrolyte concentration and its osmotic pressure are maintained within narrow limits. If this balance is disturbed in any way due to vomiting, diarrhoea or haemorrhage or any other condition leading to the accumulation or depletion of any or some of the ions, this should be rectified by administering the solution suitable for meeting the situation as given below:

1. Volume depletion (loss of sodium and water)

Here there is loss of fluid leading to dehydration. This may be caused by vomiting, diarrhoea or haemorrhage. This can be treated by using sodium chloride injection (0.9%) or balanced isotonic electrolyte solutions to restore the extracellular fluid volume.

2. Hypernatremia (loss of water in excess of sodium)

This may result from reduced intake of water or unusual water loss. Since water has been lost, there is an increase of osmotic pressure in both ECF and ICF. The best way to treat this condition is to give 5% dextrose injection to replace the water lost.

3. Hyponatremia (loss of sodium in excess of water)

This may result from conditions such as adrenocortical insufficiency, excessive sweating etc. This can be treated by giving sodium chloride injection (0.9%).

4. Oedema (volume excess)

This is due to accumulation of excess of fluid in the interstitial space with salt retention. This is seen in patients with congestive heart failure, kidney disease etc. Diuretics are used to treat this condition.

From the above discussion, it should be clear that electrolyte balance of the extracellular fluid may be disturbed at times due to various reasons and it can be restored by administering the solutions of suitable electrolytes. The most important of these electrolytes are sodium chloride and potassium chloride and their preparations.

1. SODIUM CHLORIDE, NaCl

Preparation

(a) **From Sea Water:** Sea water contains about 3 per cent of sodium chloride in addition to other substances. At high tide the sea water is allowed to flow into the shallow ponds where the less soluble material and suspended matters precipitate out. It then goes to the crystallizing pond. There it is evaporated so that the crystallized salt separates out. In the next pans, the more soluble salts such as magnesium sulphate, potassium iodide etc. are removed. The calcium and magnesium salts are removed by treating the brine with either soda ash (commercial anhydrous sodium carbonate) and lime or soda ash and caustic soda (sodium hydroxide) and allowing the precipitate to settle. The purified brine is concentrated and evaporated in triple effect evaporators.

(b) **From Underground Rock-salt Deposits:** Holes are drilled into the rock-salt beds and water is sent to run down the holes into the salt bed. The salt solution, now known as brine, is pumped to the surface and evaporated in triple effect evaporators. This is purified by a special lime soda process (refer above under method (a) and very pure sodium chloride is obtained.

(c) The purest form of salt (analytical grade) is now obtained by passing hydrogen chloride gas into a saturated solution of the salt. Very pure sodium chloride precipitates out. The crystals are centrifuged and dried.

113

Hydrogen chloride dissolves in water to form hydrochloric acid in which sodium chloride is only slightly soluble. The principle of solubility product also comes into play.

Physical Properties

Sodium chloride occurs in the form of colourless, transparent cubes or as a white, crystalline powder. It is odourless and has a saline taste. It is slightly hygroscopic possibly due to the presence of small amounts of magnesium or calcium chloride. It is freely soluble in water (1 in 2.8) and slightly soluble in alcohol.

Chemical Properties

1. Sodium chloride gives a curdy white precipitate of silver chloride with solution of silver nitrate.

$$NaCl + AgNO_3 \longrightarrow AgCl\downarrow + NaNO_3$$

The precipitate which is affected by light (i.e. photosensitive) is soluble in dilute ammonia and insoluble in nitric acid.

2. It reacts with sulphuric acid or phosphoric acid to give hydrochloric acid.

$$2NaCl + H_2SO_4 \longrightarrow 2HCl + Na_2SO_4$$

3. Sodium chloride is rather easily oxidized to liberate free chlorine. For eg. heating with manganese dioxide and concentrated sulphuric acid produces chlorine:

$$2NaCl + MnO_2 + 2H_2SO_4 \longrightarrow MnSO_4 + Na_2SO_4 + 2H_2O + Cl_2$$

Electrolytic oxidation of sodium chloride (solution of sodium chloride) is useful in the production of sodium hydroxide and chlorine (refer under sodium hydroxide). It is official in I.P.

Official Tests for Identity

Gives the reactions characteristic of sodium and of chlorides (see Chapter 13).

Standard: Contains between 99.5 and 100.5 per cent of NaCl, calculated with reference to the substance dried to constant weight at 130°C.

Storage Condition: Since it may be slightly hygroscopic due to the presence of small amounts of calcium or magnesium chloride, store in a well closed container.

Chemical Incompatibility: Sodium chloride is incompatible with certain sodium salts such as soap which consists of sodium salts of fatty acids. The soap may be precipitated out from solution by the addition of sodium chloride through the principle of solubility product coming into play .

Assay: An accurately weighed quantity is dissolved in water and a known excess of N/10 silver nitrate solution, concentrated nitric acid and nitrobenzene are added. It is titrated with N/10 ammonium thiocyanate solution using ferric ammonium sulphate as indicator.

This is a modified Volhard's method. Sodium chloride is precipitated as silver chloride by the addition of silver nitrate. Nitrobenzene is added to coagulate the silver chloride so that it will not interfere with the titration of excess of silver nitrate with N/10 ammonium thiocyanate.

Previously (in I.P.'66) sodium chloride was assayed by direct titration in neutral solution with N/10 silver nitrate using potassium chromate as indicator. The same cannot be used now since silver chromate formed at the end point is soluble in acid.

$$AgNO_3 + NaCl \longrightarrow AgCl\downarrow + NaNO_3$$

$$AgNO_3 + NH_4SCN \longrightarrow AgSCN + NH_4NO_3$$

Medicinal Uses: Electrolyte Replenisher: Sodium chloride exerts the effect of both the chloride ion and the sodium ion. Deficiency of sodium chloride leads to "salt hunger".

It is used as a fluid and electrolyte replenisher in the form of various solutions such as Sodium Chloride Hypertonic Injection, Compound Sodium Chloride Solution and Sodium Chloride and Dextrose Injection.

2. OFFICIAL PREPARATTIONS OF SODIUM CHLORIDE

The following preparations of sodium chloride are official in I.P.1985 and are used to restore fluid and electrolyte balance in the body.

(a) Sodium Chloride Injection, I.P.

This is a sterile ,isotonic solution of sodium chloride in water for injection. It contains 0.9% w/v of sodium chloride (150 millimoles each of sodium and chloride ions).

Storage: The injection should be stored in single dose containers made of glass or plastic. On keeping, small solid particles may separate in a glass container. Such an injection having such visible glass particles should not be used. A caution to this effect should be given on the label.

Medicinal Use: Fluid and electrolyte replenisher and isotonic vehicle

(b) Sodium Chloride Hypertonic Injection, I.P. (Hypertonic Saline)

This is a sterile, hypertonic solution of sodium chloride in water for injection. It contains 1.60% w/v of sodium chloride or 270 millimoles each of sodium and chloride ions per litre.

Storage: The injection should be stored in single dose containers made of glass or plastic. On keeping small solid particles may separate in a glass container. Such an injection having such visible glass particles should not be used. A caution to this effect should be given on the label.

Medicinal Use: Fluid and electrolyte replenisher: Since this is a hypertonic injection, it should be given intravenously very slowly. It is administered when there is a severe electrolyte imbalance.

(c) Compound Sodium Chloride Injection, I.P. (Ringer's Injection)

This contains 0.86% w/v of sodium chloride, 0.03% w/v of potassium chloride and 0.033% w/v of calcium chloride in water for injection, that is, it contains 147.5 mEq (millequivalents) of sodium, 4 mEq of potassium, 4.5 mEq of calcium and 156 mEq of chloride ions per litre.

Storage: The injection should be stored in single-dose containers made of glass or plastic. When it is kept in glass containers, small solid particles may separate out. A solution containing such glass particles should not be used. A caution to this effect should be given on the label.

Medicinal Use: Fluid and electrolyte replenisher.

(d) Compound Sodium Chloride Solution, I.P. (Ringer's Solution)

This solution is a sterile solution of sodium chloride, potassium chloride and calcium chloride in purified water. It contains these salts in the same proportions as in the Compound Sodium Chloride Injection I.P.

Storage: It should be stored in tightly-closed containers.

Medicinal Use: Irrigation solution for external use.

(e) Sodium Chloride and Dextrose Injection, I.P.

This is a sterile solution of sodium chloride and dextrose in water for injection. It may contain any strength of sodium chloride from 0.11% to 0.45% w/v and correspondingly from 5% to 2.5% w/v of dextrose so that the solution will be isotonic. About seven different solutions containing the quantities of sodium chloride and dextrose as given in the I.P. can be made subject to the condition that all the solutions should be isotonic.

Storage: The injection should be stored in single-dose containers in a cool place. Small solid particles may separate on keeping and such an injection should not be used . A caution to this effect should be given on the label.

Medicinal Use: Fluid nutrient and electrolyte replenisher: If the patient is also weak and his nutritional status is to be toned up, this injection containing dextrose in addition to sodium chloride may be given.

3. POTASSIUM CHLORIDE, KCl

Preparation

1. It is extracted from natural minerals such as carnallite and sylvite. Carnallite is $MgCl_2$. KCl. $6H_2O$, whereas sylvite is a mixture of sodium and potassium chlorides. Potassium chloride is extracted from carnallite by using a process of fractional crystallisation.

2. In the laboratory it is prepared by the action of hydrochloric acid on either potassium carbonate or potassium bicarbonate.

$$K_2CO_3 + 2HCl \longrightarrow 2KCl + H_2O + CO_2\uparrow$$
$$KHCO_3 + HCl \longrightarrow KCl + H_2O + CO_2\uparrow$$

Physical and Chemical Properties

Potassium chloride consists of colourless, prismatic or cubical crystals or occurs as a white, granular powder. It is odourless and has a saline taste. It is freely soluble in cold or hot water. It is practically insoluble in alcohol and ether. Its aqueous solution is neutral to litmus.

As for chemical properties, it undergoes almost the same reactions as sodium chloride. It precipitates silver chloride, lead chloride and mercurous chloride when treated with soluble silver, lead and mercurous salts. It is official in I.P.

Official Tests for Identity

A solution of potassium chloride in water gives the reactions of potassium and of chlorides (see Chapter 13).

Standard: Potassium chloride contains not less than 99 per cent of KCl, calculated with reference to the dried substance.

Storage Condition: Since it is quite stable in air, it is enough if it is stored in well-closed containers.

Chemical Incompatibility: It is incompatible with soluble mercurous, silver and lead salts precipitating their chlorides.

Medicinal Use: Electrolyte replenisher.

It is used along with sodium chloride and calcium chloride in Compound Sodium Chloride Injection, I.P. (Ringer's Injection) and Compound Sodium Chloride Solution I.P. (Ringer's Solution) for restoring electrolyte balance. However potassium chloride solution irritates the gastric mucosa and may cause ulceration. So it must be well diluted before oral administration. It is also used as a diuretic and to treat hypopotassaemia (depletion of potassium in the body).

4. OFFICIAL PREPARATIONS OF POTASSIUM CHLORIDE

The following are the official preparations of potassium chloride:-

1. Compound Sodium Chloride Injection, I.P.
2. Compound Sodium Chloride Solution, I.P.

ACID-BASE BALANCE

The pH of the arterial blood is maintained at 7.4 and the pH of the venous blood and interstitial fluid at 7.35. If the pH falls below 7.0 or rises above 7.8, the person concerned will die. Generally if the pH of the ECF goes below 7.4 the condition is known as acidosis and if it goes above 7.4 it is known as alkalosis. The acid base balance is a dynamic equilibrium and it is maintained by three factors:

1. Action of chemical buffers present in the blood such as carbonic acid and sodium bicarbonate.

2. Respiration which constantly removes carbon dioxide from the body.

3. Excretion through kidney of acid as well as base.

Potassium

Potassium is the major intracellular cation. It is also present in plasma in a concentration from 3.4 to 5.6 mEq/1. Potassium is necessary for muscle contraction, enzyme action, nerve conduction and cell membrane function. It is also necessary for the proper functioning of the heart. Treatment with diuretics is the most common cause of hypokalaemia or depletion of potassium in the body. It is treated by giving potassium chloride which should be administered cautiously. Compound Sodium Chloride Injection, I.P. is used when other ions such as sodium and chloride (other than potassium) have also to be supplemented.

The following are the electrolytes used for maintaining the physiological acid-base balance.

1. SODIUM ACETATE, CH_3COONa, $3H_2O$

Preparation: Sodium acetate is prepared by neutralising acetic acid with either sodium bicarbonate or sodium carbonate. The solution is filtered and evaporated to crystallisation.

$$CH_3COOH + NaHCO_3 \longrightarrow CH_3COONa + H_2O + CO_2\uparrow$$

$$2CH_3COOH + Na_2CO_3 \longrightarrow 2CH_3COONa + H_2O + CO_2\uparrow$$

Physical and Chemical Properties

Sodium acetate occurs either as colourless crystals or as a white, granular powder. It is either odourless or has a slight acetous odour. It has a slightly saline and bitter taste. It is very soluble in water. When exposed to warm, dry air, it effloresces. Along with acetic acid, it acts as a buffer. When sodium acetate is heated, it dissolves in its own water of crystallization. On further heating the water is removed and it becomes solid. By careful heating to prevent charring, it is melted and may be poured into a clean surface. The product now obtained is known as 'fused sodium acetate' which is used for some acetylation reactions.

When a mineral acid is added to sodium acetate, acetic acid is formed and the smell of vinegar is noticed.

$$CH_3COONa + HCl \longrightarrow CH_3COOH + NaCl$$

$$2CH_3COONa + H_2SO_4 \longrightarrow 2CH_3COOH + Na_2SO_4$$

Sodium acetate, warmed with sulphuric acid and ethyl alcohol, gives ethyl acetate whcih has a fruity odour.

$$CH_3COOH + C_2H_5OH \xrightarrow{H_2SO_4} CH_3COOC_2H_5 + H_2O$$

When sodium acetate is ignited (heated very strongly), it is converted into sodium carbonate.

$$2CH_3COONa,3H_2O + 4O_2 \xrightarrow{\Delta} Na_2CO_3 + 6H_2O + 3CO_2\uparrow$$

It gives a deep red colour with neutral ferric chloride. Ferric acetate is formed.

$$FeCl_3 + 3CH_3COONa \rightleftharpoons (CH_3COO)_3Fe + 3NaCl$$

It is official in I.P.

Official Tests for Identity: Sodium acetate gives the reactions of sodium and of acetates (see Chapter 13).

Non-Official Tests for Identity

1. Heat the substance in a test tube. It becomes liquid and then becomes solid. Finally it fuses at a high temperature. It emits

non-inflammable vapours and leaves a residue of sodium carbonate and carbon. The residue answers the test for sodium and gives effervescence with acids.

2. When the solution of the substance is added to Ferric Chloride T.S., a deep red colour is produced.

Standard: Sodium Acetate should contain between 99 per cent and 101 per cent of $C_2H_3NaO_2,3H_2O$.

Storage Condition: Since it effloresces in warm, dry air, store it in tightly closed containers.

Chemical Incompatibility: Since an aqueous solution of sodium acetate is slightly alkaline, it is incompatible with acids. However in combination with acetic acid, it acts as a good buffer.

Medicinal Uses: When sodium acetate is given orally, it is absorbed and oxidized in the body to give sodium bicarbonate. So it is useful as a **diuretic, urinary alkalizer and systemic alkalizer.** It is also useful for preparing peritoneal dialysis fluids.

2. POTASSIUM ACETATE, CH₃COOK

Preparation: Potassium acetate is prepared by neutralizing acetic acid with either potassium bicarbonate or potassium carbonate until effervescence ceases. The solution is evaporated to dryness and fused. While the mass is still warm, it is reduced to powder and bottled.

$$CH_3COOH + KHCO_3 \longrightarrow CH_3COOK + H_2O + CO_2\uparrow$$

Physical and Chemical Properties: Potassium acetate occurs either as colourless crystals or as a white, crystalline powder. It is odourless. However it may have a slight acetous odour especially when it is damp. It is deliquescent which means that it absorbs moisture very rapidly when it is exposed to air and also dissolves in the water absorbed to form a solution. It is very soluble in water.

Like sodium acetate, potassium acetate also, on strong ignition, evolves volatile, non-inflammable vapours and leaves a residue of potassium carbonate and carbon.

$$2CH_3COOK + 4O_2 \xrightarrow{\Delta} K_2CO_3 + 3H_2O + 3CO_2\uparrow$$

The residue is alkaline to litmus and answers tests for potassium. It also gives effervescence with acids. It is official in B.P. 1988.

Official Tests for Identity: Potassium acetate gives the reactions characteristic of potassium, and of acetates (see Chapter 13).

Standard: Potassium acetate should contain between 99 per cent and 101 per cent of $C_2H_3O_2K$, calculated with reference to the dried substance.

Storage Condition: Since it is very deliquescent, store in tightly closed containers.

Chemical Incompatibility: Like sodium acetate an aqueous solution of potassium acetate also is slightly alkaline and so is incompatible with acids.

Medicinal Uses: Like sodium acetate, it is also converted into bicarbonate in the body. So it acts as a **diuretic and urinary alkalizer.** It is also used in solutions for haemodialysis and peritoneal dialysis.

3. SODIUM BICARBONATE , NaHCO₃

Refer Chapter 4.

SODIUM BICARBONATE INJECTION

This is official as Sodium Bicarbonate Intravenous Infusion in B.P.1988. It is a sterile solution of sodium bicarbonate in water for injection. Intravenous infusions containing 1.26, 1.4, 2.74, 4.2, 5.0 and 8.4% w/v of sodium bicarbonate are available. A preparation containing 1.4% w/v of sodium bicarbonate contains 167 millimoles each of sodium and bicarbonate ions. It is sterilised by heating in an autoclave. Containers containing visible particles should not be used.

Medicinal Use: Systemic alkalizer. The injection is administered intravenously to raise the pH of the blood in acidosis due to diabetes mellitus and certain other diseases.

4. SODIUM CITRATE, Na₃C₆H₅O₇.2H₂O

Preparation: Sodium citrate is prepared by reacting a solution of citric acid with either sodium carbonate or sodium bicarbonate. The effervescence is allowed to subside and the solution is evaporated to crystallization.

$$3NaHCO_3 + H_3C_6H_5O_7 \cdot H_2O \longrightarrow Na_3C_6H_5O_7 \cdot 2H_2O$$

         Citric acid   Sod.citrate $+2H_2O + 3CO_2\uparrow$

Physical and Chemical Properties

Sodium citrate consists of white, granular crystals or occurs as a white crystalline powder. It is odourless and has a cool, saline taste. It is slightly deliquescent in moist air but effloresces slowly in dry air. It is freely soluble in cold water and very soluble in boiling water. It is slightly alkaline in aqueous solution.

When heated, it starts to lose water at about $100^{\circ}C$ and becomes anhydrous at about $150^{\circ}C$. On strong heating, it carbonizes evolving non-inflammable gases with a pungent acrid odour and leaving a residue of sodium bicarbonate.

$$2Na_3C_6H_5O_7, 2H_2O + 9O_2 \xrightarrow{\Delta} 3Na_2CO_3 + 5H_2O + 9CO_2\uparrow$$

Sodium ctirate is the salt of a strong base with a weak acid, that is, citric acid which is a tricarboxylic hydroxy acid.

$$
\begin{array}{l}
CH_2COOH \\
| \\
C(OH)COOH + 3NaOH \longrightarrow \\
| \\
CH_2COOH
\end{array}
\qquad
\begin{array}{l}
CH_2COONa \\
| \\
C(OH)COONa2H_2O + H_2O \\
| \\
CH_2COONa
\end{array}
$$

            or $Na_3C_6H_5O_7 \cdot 2H_2O$

                 Sodium citrate

Because of the presence of the alcoholic hydroxyl group, sodium citrate possesses the property of sequestration or complexation. When added to blood, it sequesters the blood calcium as an undissociated organic complex and thus the coagulation of blood is prevented. Sodium citrate is official in B.P.1988.

Official Tests for Identity: A solution in carbon dioxide–free water gives the reactions characteristic of sodium salts and of citrates (see Chapter 13).

Standard: Sodium Citrate contains between 99 and 101 per cent of $Na_3C_6H_5O_7$, calculated with reference to the anhydrous substance.

Storage Condition: Since it deliquesces in moist air and effloresces in dry air, it must be kept in a tightly closed or airtight container.

Chemical Incompatibility: Since it complexes metallic ions such as ferrous iron, ferric iron, calcium etc., to that extent it is incompatible with the solutions containing them and does not allow the metallic ions to undergo the reactions meant for them since the metallic ions are not in the free state but complexed into undissociated organic complexes.

Medicinal and Pharmaceutical Uses: Systemic alkalizer and diuretic. Sodium citrate is oxidized in the body to sodium bicarbonate. It is also used as an **anticoagulant.**

5. POTASSIUM CITRATE, $K_3C_6H_5O_7$. H_2O

Preparation: Potassium citrate is prepared in the same way as sodium citrate by neutralizing a solution of citric acid with either potassium carbonate or potassium bicarbonate. The effervescence is allowed to subside and the solution is evaporated to crystallization.

$$3KHCO_3 + H_3C_6H_5O_7.\, H_2O \longrightarrow K_3C_6H_5O_7\, .H_2O + 3CO_2\uparrow$$
$$\text{Potassium citrate} \quad + 3H_2O$$

Physical and Chemical Properties

Potassium citrate occurs as transparant crystals or as a white granular powder. It is odourless and has a cooling, saline taste. It is hygroscopic and very soluble in water.

When heated, potassium citrate begins to lose water at $100^{0}C$ and becomes anhydrous at about $200^{0}C$. On further strong heating, it carbonizes and evolves non-inflammable gases having a pungent, acrid odour. It leaves a residue of carbon and potassium carbonate which can be tested by adding dilute acid (effervescence).

$$2K_3C_6H_5O_7.\, H_2O + 9O_2 \longrightarrow 3K_2CO_3 + 9CO_2\uparrow + 6H_2O$$

It is official in I.P.

Standard: Potassium citrate contains between 99 and 101 per cent of $K_3C_6H_5O_7$, calculated with reference to the anhydrous substance.

Storage Condition: Since it is hygroscopic, it must be stored in a tightly closed or airtight contianer.

Chemical Incompatibility: Same as for sodium citrate.

Medicinal and Pharmaceutical Uses: Systemic alkalizer, diuretic, expectorant and diaphoretic.

SODIUM LACTATE

Sodium lactate is a colourless thick liquid without odour. It is soluble in water. Usually it is available as a 70 to 80 per cent solution in water. It has the following structure:

$$
\begin{array}{c}
CH_3 \diagdown \qquad \diagup H \\
C \\
HO \diagup \qquad \diagdown COONa
\end{array}
$$

Since the central carbon atom is asymmetric, two stereoisomeric forms of D-lactate and L-Lactate are available. The racemic mixture (combination of both D-and L-forms) is present in the injection. The L-lactate is converted in the body to sodium bicarbonate and so acts as a systemic alkalizer. In the I.P. racemic sodium lactate is made in the preparation of injection by reacting lactic acid with sodium hydroxide.

6. SODIUM LACTATE INJECTION

Preparation: This is an one-sixth molar solution which is approximately isotonic with blood serum. It is prepared by reacting sodium hydroxide and lactic acid and heating in an autocalave at $115^{\circ}C$ to $116^{\circ}C$ for one hour. By heating at a very high temperature it is possible to ensure that the lactic anhydride is fully hydrolysed to lactic acid which then reacts with sodium hydroxide along with the already present free lactic acid. Then the pH is adjusted to a value of 5 to 7 with phenol red solution and the solution is made up to volume. It is filtered and immediately sterilised by heating in an autoclave.

Sodium Lactate Injection is a clear, colourless solution and it is official in I.P.

Official Tests for Identity

1. When the injection is warmed with potassium permanganate, it gives off acetaldehyde which can be recognised by its characteristic odour.

2. The injection is evaporated to dryness. The residue gives the reactions of sodium (refer Chapter 13).

Standard: Sodium lactate injection contains about 1.85 per cent w/v of $C_3H_5NaO_3$(sodium lactate). (The injection is one-sixth molar and contains approcimately 167 millimoles of sodium and lactate)

Storage Condition: Should be stored only in single-dose containers of glass or plastic. On keeping, there may be separation of small particles in glass containers. So a caution should be given on the label that the injection should not be used if it contains visible particles.

Medicinal Use: Fluid and electrolyte replenisher. It is easily oxidised to sodium bicarbonate and so acts as a **systemic alkalizer**. Its advantages over sodium bicarbonate are that it can be readily sterilise and also that it does not produce systemic alkalosis like sodium bicarbonate.

7. AMMONIUM CHLORIDE, NH₄Cl

Refer Chapter 8.

AMMONIUM CHLORIDE INJECTION

Ammonium chloride injection is not official now. However it can be used as a **systemic acidifier** by injecting a 2% solution along with glucose. It acts by reducing the alkali reserve in the body and so is useful in reducing metabolic alkalosis. If it is given in large doses, it makes the urine acidic and acts as a diuretic also.

COMBINATION OF ORAL ELECTROLYTE POWDERS AND SOLUTIONS

In cholera there is a masive diarrohea with watery stools and also vomiting resulting in a marked depletion of sodium, potassium and bicarbonate leading to metabolic acidosis. Hence it is necessary to make good the water loss (dehydration) and electrolyte loss and correct the acidosis in addition to treatment with antibiotics etc. Even in cases of severe diarrhoea (other than cholera), it may become necessary to correct the dehydration and electrolyte depletion. Normally this condition is treated with isotonic saline and isotonic sodium bicarbonate solution given intravenously.

Now it has been found that where facilities for intravenous therapy are not available, an oral glucose-electrolyte solution may be given and serves equally well. Addition of glucose to the electrolyte solution enhances the sodium and water absorption by the small intestine. This Oral Rehydration Therapy (O.R.T) has several advantages:

1. The oral treatment is very cheap, much cheaper than the intravenous solution.

2. No expertise is needed to give this by mouth. It can be given by anybody.

3. It is not necessary that the solution should be sterile.

4. Vomiting is easily corrected by the therapy itself.

5. Patients strong enough to drink take this easily.

The W.H.O has recommended the following formula for oral rehydration therapy (O.R.T):

Sodium chloride	3.5 g
Potasssium chloride	1.5 g
Sodium bicarbonate	2.5 g
Glucose (Anhydrous Dextrose,I.P.)	20.0 g
Boiled water to make	100 ml

This contains sodium 90 mEq/l, potassium 20mEq/l, chloride 80 mEq/l and bicarbonate 30 mEq/l. The constitutents are mixed and supplied in sealed packets in the form of a ready to dissolve powder.

This formula may be slightly varied by including sodium citrate in place of sodium bicarbonate.

Sodium chloride	3.5 g
Potassium chloride	1.5 g
Sodium citrate	2.9 g
Dexrose (anhydrous)	20.0 g

The powder may be dissolved in boiled water and made upto one litre which is equivalent to 5 tumbler fulls (200 ml each). It contains the same proportions of electrolytes as in the previous formula except that this powder contains 9.9 mEq/l of citrate in place of the bicarbonate.

DOSAGE: Depending upon age and severity of dehydration.

Infants and Children: 1-2 litres (5-10 glasses) over a period of 24 hours.

Adults: 2-4 litres (10-20 glasses) over a period of 24 hours.

Sucrose may be used in place of glucose (dextrose) with equally good results. Starch or rice powder may also be used. We may recall here that our people have beeen using rice conjee as diet for patients suffering from diarrhoea.

In the light of the above, a recently recommended method is to dissolve one pinch of salt and two teaspoons of sugar in a tumbler full of water and give it to the patient making the O.R.T., even simpler.

CHAPTER 10

INORGANIC OFFICIAL COMPOUNDS OF IRON, IODINE AND CALCIUM

I. INORGANIC OFFICIAL COMPOUNDS OF IRON

The following iron compounds are official in I.P.:-

1. Ferrous fumarate
2. Ferrous gluconate
3. Ferrous sulphate
4. Dried ferrous sulphate
5. Iron and ammonium citrate

1. FERROUS FUMARATE, $\left[\begin{array}{c} HC\,COO^- \\ \parallel \\ {}^-OOC\,CH \end{array} \right] Fe^{2+}$ or $C_4H_2FeO_4$

Preparation: Ferrous fumarate is prepared by treating ferrous sulphate with sodium fumarate.

Physical and Chemical Properties

Ferrous fumarate is a reddish orange to reddish brown fine powder. It may contain soft lumps which produce a yellow streak when crushed. It has a slight odour and a slightly astringent taste. It is slightly soluble in water.

It answers the tests for ferrous iron and for fumarate ion. It is assayed by titration with ceric ammonium sulphate using ferroin sulphate solution as indicator. Here the ferrous fumarate is oxidised. It is official in I.P.

Official Tests for Identity

1. A small quantity of the sample is heated with diluted hydrochloric acid on a water bath for fifteen minutes, cooled and filtered. The filtrate gives the reactions of ferrous salts (see Chapter 13).

2. The precipitate obtained in (1) above is washed with a mixture of dilute hydrochloric acid and dried. It is suspended in sodium carbonate solution and potassium permanganate solution is added drop by drop. The permanganate is decolourised and a brownish solution is obtained.

3. A small quantity of the sample is mixed with resorcinol, a few drops of concentrated sulphuric acid are added and gently heated. A deep red, semisolid mass is obtained. It is added to a large volume of water. An orange-yellow solution without any fluorescence is obtained.

Standard: Ferrous Fumarate contains not less than 93 per cent of $C_4H_2FeO_4$ calculated with reference to the dried substance.

Storage Condition: Store in a well-closed container.

Chemical Incompatibility: It is quite stable to oxidation or hydrolysis. However since it is a ferrous salt and also a fumarate with a double bond in the structure, it is incompatible with strong oxidising agents.

Medicinal Use: Haematinic. It is useful in the prevention and treatment of iron-deficinecy anaemias.

2. FERROUS GLUCONATE, $[CH_2OH(CHOH)_4COO]_2$ Fe. $2H_2O$

Preparation: Glucose is oxidised by bacterial fermentation to gluconic acid. The gluconic acid so obtained is treated with ferrous carbonate to give ferrous gluconate. It is crystallized out with 2 molecules of water of hydration and dried.

$$C_6H_{12}O_6 \longrightarrow HC_6H_{11}O_7$$

Glucose   Gluconic acid

$$2HC_6H_{11}O_7 + FeCO_3 + H_2O \longrightarrow Fe(C_6H_{11}O_7)_2. 2H_2O + CO_2\uparrow$$

Gluconic   Ferrous   Ferrous gluconate
acid   carbonate

Physical and Chemical Properties

Ferrous gluconate occurs as yellowish-grey or pale greenish-yellow, fine powder or granules. It has a slight odour like that of burnt sugar. It is fairly soluble in cold water and more soluble in warm water.

An aqueous solution is acid in reaction and it answers the reactions of ferrous salts and of the gluconate ion. It is assayed by titration with ceric ammonium sulphate solution like ferrous fumarate

It is official in I.P.

Official Tests for Identity

1. A solution of the sample in water gives the reactions of ferrous salts (see Chapter 13).

2. To a small quantity of the sample are added water, glacial acetic acid and freshly distilled phenylhydrazine. The mixture is heated on a water bath for thirty minutes. It is cooled and the inner surface of the test tube is scratched with a glass rod until crystals of gluconic acid phenylhydrazide begin to form. After setting aside for ten minutes it is filtered. The precipitate is dissolved in hot water mixed with a small amount of decolourising charcoal and filtered in to a test tube. The filtrate is cooled and the inner surface of the test tube is scratched. White crystals of pure gluconic acid phenylhydrazide are obtained. They melt at about $202^{\circ}C$ with decomposition.

Standard: Ferrous gluconate contains not less than 95 per cent of $C_{12}H_{22}FeO_{14}$ calculated with reference to the dried substance.

Storage Condition: Since it is affected by light, store in well closed, light resistant containers.

Chemical Incompatibility: It is incompatible with oxidizing agents.

Medicinal Use: Haematinic. It is useful in the prevention and treatment of iron-deficiency anaemias.

3. FERROUS SULPHATE, $FeSO_4,7H_2O$.

Preparation: It is prepared by dissolving a slight excess of iron in dilute sulphuric acid and concentrating to get green crystals of ferrous sulphate.

$$Fe + H_2SO_4 \longrightarrow FeSO_4 + H_2\uparrow$$

On the manufacturing scale scrap iron is used.

Physical and Chemical Properties: This is crystalline ferrous sulphate containing seven molcules of water of hydration. It occurs in the form of transparent, green crystals or as a pale bluish-green, crystalline powder. It is odourless and has a metallic, astringent taste. It effloresces in dry air. When exposed to moist air, it is slowly oxidised and is coated with a brown, basic ferric sulphate. When this takes place, the sample should not be used. It is soluble in water and practically insoluble in alcohol. Ferrous sulphate combines with alkali sulphates to form double salts. Ferrous ammonium sulphate, $FeSO_4(NH_4)_2SO_4 . 6H_2O$, is one such. It is used in analytical chemistry.

Ferrous sulphate is oxidised by acidified potassium permanganate to ferric sulphate. This is used as the assay method for estimating ferrous sulphate. Ferrous sulphate is official in I.P.

Official Tests for Identity: Gives the reactions characteristic of ferrous salts and sulphates (refer Chapter 13).

Standard: Contains not less than 98 per cent and not more than the equivalent of 105 per cent of $FeSO_4 . 7H_2O$.

Storage Condition: Since it effloresces in dry air and is oxidised in moist air, store in tightly closed containers.

Chemical Incompatibility: Since it is a ferrous salt, it is incompatible with oxidising agents. It is also incompatible with tannin containing preparations.

1. Assay (I.P.1985)

An accurately weighed quantity is dissolved in a mixture of water and dilute sulphuric acid. Then it is titrated with N/10 ceric ammonium sulphate using ferroin sulphate as indicator.

Ferrous sulphate is oxidised to ferric sulphate by the ceric ammonium sulphate. The indicator ferroin sulphate solution is nothing but orthophenanthroline ferrous complex. The end point is marked by the appearance of a light blue colour.

2. Assay (I.P.'66)

An accurately weighed quantity is dissolved in dilute sulphuric acid and titrated against N/10 potassium permanganate. In this way ferrous sulphate is oxidised by the nascent oxygen from the acidified potassium permanganate to ferric sulphate. Potassium permanganate acts as its own indicator. Appearance of pale pink colour is the end point.

$$2KMnO_4 + 3H_2SO_4 \longrightarrow K_2SO_4 + 2MnSO_4 + 3H_2O + 5(O)$$

$$2FeSO_4 + H_2SO_4 + O \longrightarrow Fe_2(SO_4)_3 + H_2O$$

Ferrous   Ferric
sulphate   sulphate

or $10FeSO_4 + 2KMnO_4 + 8H_2SO_4 \longrightarrow 5Fe_2(SO_4)_3 + 2MnSO_4$
$$+ K_2SO_4 + H_2O$$

Medicinal Use: Haematinic. This is the most popular of the ferrous salts and also the cheapest.

4. DRIED FERROUS SULPHATE

This is a greyish white to buff-coloured powder with a metallic astringent taste. It dissolves slowly but completely in water. Otherwise it resembles Ferrous Sulphate.

Preparation: It is prepared by drying the crystalline salt in an oven at 40°C till it loses the correct amount of water. It is a mixture of hydrates and corresponds to the formula $FeSO_4 . 2H_2O$. It must be immediately put into a bottle and tightly stoppered.

Official Tests for Identity: Same as for Ferrous Sulphate.

Standard: Contains not less than 80 per cent and not more than 90 per cent of $FeSO_4$.

Chemical Incompatibility: Same as for Ferrous Sulphate.

Storage Condition: Store in a well-closed container.

Medicinal Use: Haematinic. Pharmaceutical aid.

5. IRON AND AMMONIUM CITRATE
(FERRIC AMMONIUM CITRATE)

Preparation: This can be considered in stages as given below:

1. **Preparation of Ferric Hydroxide:** Ferric hydroxide is prepared by the interaction between a ferric salt solution and an alkali such as ammonia, sodium hydroxide or sodium carbonate. The ferric salt solution should be added to the alkali with stirring and not vice versa. Ferric hydroxide is precipitated and it is collected by filtration and washed.

$$Fe_2(SO_4)_3 + 6NaOH \longrightarrow 2Fe(OH)_3 + 3Na_2SO_4$$
Ferric sulphate   Ferric hydroxide

2. **Preparation of Ferric Citrate:** Citric acid is added to the wet precipitate (which is not dried) to dissolve nearly the whole of the precipitate.

$$Fe(OH)_3 + H_3C_6H_5O_7 \longrightarrow FeC_6H_5O_7 + 3H_2O$$
Citric acid   Ferric citrate

3. Preparation of Ferric Ammonium Citrate

(a) Formation of Ferric Ammonium Citrate: A slight excess of ammonia is added and any undissolved ferric hydroxide is removed by filtration.

(b) Concentration: The filtrate is clear and reddish brown in colour. It is evaporated to a syrup, adding ammonia from time to time so that an excess of ammonia is maintained throughout the evaporation process.

(c) Scaling: Finally the syrup is painted on glass plates and dried below $40^\circ C$. Then it is scrapped off as scales (reddish brown). Green scales are obtained if excess of citric acid is used.

Physical and Chemical Properties: Iron and Ammonium Citrate is a complex ammonium ferric citrate. It occurs as thin, transparent, dark-red scales or granules or as a brownish red granular powder.

It is odourless and has an astringent taste. It deliquesces in air and is affected by light. It is very soluble in water and almost insoluble in alcohol. An aqueous solution does not give the normal reactions for iron. Only after acidification with hydrochloric acid, it gives the reactions for iron.

There is a view that ferric ammonium citrate is a solid sol of a basic colloidal complex $FeC_6H_5O_7.2Fe(OH)_3$ dispersed in ammonium citrate. It is assayed by treating with acidified potassium iodide. The acid releases the ferric iron in the ferric ammonium citrate and the ferric iron then oxidises the potassium iodide to iodine which is estimated by titration against standard sodium thiosulphate solution.

$$2FeCl_3 + 2KI \longrightarrow I_2 + 2FeCl_2 + 2KCl$$

$$I_2 + 2Na_2S_2O_3 \longrightarrow 2NaI + Na_2S_4O_6$$

Ferric Ammonium citrate is official in I.P.

Official Tests for Identity

1. Ignite gently and dissolve the residue in hydrochloric acid. The solution gives the reactions characteristic of ferric salts (see Chapter 13).

2. Warm with solution of sodium hydroxide. Ammonia is evolved and the solution gives the reactions characteristic of citrates (refer Chapter 13).

Storage Condition: Since it deliquesces in moist air and is also affected by light, store in tightly closed, light resistant containers.

Chemical Incompatibility: Since the iron is in the organic form, no chemical incompatibility is usually present. However if acid is present, a ferric salt such as ferric chloride is formed and the incompatibility associated with ferric salts is now apparent. Under these conditions it is incompatible with reducing agents and also tannin–containing compounds.

Medicinal Use: Haematinic. Because of its high solubility in water, it can be used in the form of syrups, elixirs ets.

II. INORGANIC OFFICIAL COMPOUNDS OF IODINE

The following inorganic compounds are official in I.P.(I.P.1985):

1. Iodine
2. Potassium iodide

1. IODINE: Refer Chapter 5.

2. POTASSIUM IODIDE: Refer Chapter 8.

III. INORGANIC OFFICIAL COMPOUNDS OF CALCIUM

The following inorganic compounds of calcium are official in I.P.:

1. Calcium carbonate
2. Calcium chloride
3. Calcium gluconate
4. Calcium hydroxide
5. Dibasic calcium phosphate
6. Tribasic calcium phosphate

1. CALCIUM CARBONATE: Refer Chapter 14

2. CALCIUM CHLORIDE, $CaCl_2.2H_2O$

Preparation: The hexahydrate is prepared first by adding a slight excess of pure calcium carbonate to hot, diluted hydrochloric acid and filtering after the effervescence ceases. The mixture is evaporated to a syrup and allowed to crystallize at a temperature below $10^{\circ}C$. The crystals are separated by suction and put into stoppered bottles. When this hexahydrate is heated to $200^{\circ}C$ it forms the dihydrate.

$$CaCO_3 + 2HCl + 6H_2O \longrightarrow CaCl_2. 6H_2O + CO_2\uparrow + H_2O$$

Physical and Chemical Properties: Calcium chloride occurs as a white, crystalline powder or as hard fragments or granules. It is odourless and has a sharp, bitter, saline taste. It is deliquescent, that is, it absorbs moisture from the air rapidly and dissolves in the water forming a solution. It is freely soluble in cold water and very soluble in boiling water.

Calcium chloride normally forms several hydrates such as the monohydrate ($CaCl_2.H_2O$), the dihydrate ($CaCl_2.2H_2O$), the tetra hydrate ($CaCl_2.4H_2O$), and the hexahydrate ($CaCl_2.6H_2O$). All the hydrates lose water when heated and form a porous mass with variable water content. This porous mass, commonly but erroneously known as fused calcium chloride, is used for drying gases and liquids. Since it forms crystalline compounds with alcohols and ammonia gas, it is unsuitable to serve as drying agent for them. It is official in I.P.

Official Tests for Identity: An aqueous solution of the substance gives the reactions of calcium and of chlorides (refer Chapter 13).

Standard: Calcium Chloride contains between 97 and 103 per cent of $CaCl_2, 2H_2O$.

Storage Condition: Since it is very deliquescent and absorbs moisture from the atmosphere, store in tightly closed containers.

Chemical Incompatibility: Calcium salts are incompatible with sodium bicarbonate. They react with it evolving carbon dioxide. The calcium bicarbonate first formed decomposes to the carbonate evolving carbon dioxide. Calcium chloride is also incompatible with soluble alkalis forming sparingly soluble calcium hydroxide or calcium carbonate.

Medicinal Use: Calcium replenisher. It is used in combination with sodium chloride and potassium chloride in Compound Sodium Chloride Injection, I.P. (Ringer's Injection) and Compound Sodium Chloride Solution, I.P. (Ringer's Solution).

3. CALCIUM GLUCONATE, $[HOCH_2(CHOH)_4COO]_2Ca. H_2O$

Preparation: Calcium gluconate may be prepared by the oxidation of glucose to gluconic acid in the presence of calcium carbonate. The oxidation may be carried out either by bromine or by electrolytic oxidation with sodium bromide. An alternative method will be to prepare the gluconic acid first and then react it with calcium carbonate in boiling condition.

$$2HOCH_2 — (CHOH)_4 — COOH + CaCO_3 \longrightarrow$$
$$\text{Gluconic acid} \quad [HOCH_2 — (CHOH)_4 — COO]_2Ca$$
$$\text{Cal.gluconate}$$
$$+ CO_2 \uparrow + H_2O$$

Physical and Chemical Properties: Calcium gluconate occurs as a white, crystalline or granular powder. It is tasteless and odourless. It is stable in air. It loses its water of crystallisation with decomposition above $100^{\circ}C$. It is soluble in cold water, freely soluble in boiling water and insoluble in ethyl alcohol, chloroform and solvent ether.

Calcium gluconate is decomposed by mineral acids to form gluconic acid which on dehydration forms the D-gluconolactone.

$$[HOCH_2 — (CHOH)_4COO]_2 \, Ca \; + 2HCl$$

Cal.gluconate

$\downarrow$

$$HOCH_2 \, (CHOH)_4 \; COOH \; + CaCl_2$$

Gluconic acid

$\downarrow -H_2O$

$$HOCH_2 \, CHOH — CH — (CHOH)_2 — C = O$$
$$\underline{\qquad\qquad\quad O \qquad\quad}$$

D-Gluconolactone

Calcium gluconate is official in I.P.

Official Tests for Identity

1. Gives the reactions characteristic of calcium (see Chapter 13).

2. To a solution of the substance in water ferric chloride solution is added. A yellow colour is produced.

3. An aqueous solution of the substance is warmed with glacial acetic acid and phenylhydrazine. The mixture is heated on a water bath and allowed to cool. When the inside of the test tube is scratched with glass rod, crystals of gluconic acid phenylhydrazide form. They are decolourised with decolourising charcoal and dried. They melt at about $200^{\circ}C$ with decomposition.

Standard: Contains not less than 98 per cent and not more than the equivalent of 102 per cent of $C_{12}H_{22}O_{14}Ca, H_2O$.

Storage Condition: Store in well-closed container.

Chemical Incompatibility: Same as for calcium chloride

Assay: This is a complexometric assay. An accurately weighed quantity is dissolved in warm water and a definite quantity of 0.05 M magnesium sulphate solution and strong ammonia-ammonium chloride solution are added. The mixture is titrated with M/20 disodium ethylenediaminetetra acetate (EDTA or disodium salt of ethylenediaminetetraacetic acid or sodium edetate) using mordant black mixture as indicator. A blank titration taking only the quantity of 0.05M magnesium sulphate solution is done and this blank titre value is subtracted from the titre value earlier obtained for the assay.

The buffer of strong ammonia-ammonium chloride solution is added to raise and maintain the pH at 10, because at this pH only complexation takes place. Magnesium is added to give the indicator action, since the indicator does not give the wine red colour with calcium but only with magnsium. First calcium is complexed by EDTA and finally magnesium. The end point is the appearance of blue colour.The complexation of calcium by EDTA is given below:

Calcium - EDTA Complex

Medicinal and Pharmaceutical Use: Electrolyte replenisher. Calcium gluconate is administered in the form of tablets or injection in case of calcium deficiency.

4. CALCIUM HYDROXIDE: Refer Chapter 2.

5. DIBASIC CALCIUM PHOSPHATE: Refer Chapter 6.

6. TRIBASIC CALCIUM PHOSPHATE, $Ca_3(PO_4)_2$

Preparation: Tribasic calcium phosphate is prepared by the reaction between calcium chloride and secondary sodium phosphate in the presence of ammonia:

$$3CaCl_2 + 2Na_2HPO_4 + 2NH_4OH \longrightarrow Ca_3(PO_4)_2 + 4NaCl + 2NH_4Cl + 2H_2O$$

Secondary sodium phosphate   Ammonia   Tribasic calcium phosphate

The white precipitate is washed with water until free from chloride and dried at 100°C.

Physical and Chemical Properties: Tribasic calcium phosphate consists of a varible mixture of normal, basic and acid calcium phosphates. It contains calcium equivalent to not less than 90 per cent of $Ca_3(PO_4)_2$ (tribasic calcium phosphate), calculated with reference to the ignited substance.

It is a bulky , white, amorphous or microcrystalline powder, it is odourless and insoluble in water and alcohol. It readily dissolves in dilute nitric acid and in dilute hydrochloric acid. It dissolves in solutions of salts and also in a solution of carbon dioxide. Alkalis precipitate it from an acid solution. Since it is almost completely insoluble in water, it undergoes few chemical reactions. However it acts as an antacid through an interesting mechanism.It ionizes slightly in contact with water even though it is insoluble in water. The phosphate ion, being a strong base, combines with hydrogen ions (from the hydrochloric acid secreted in the stomach). It also combines with water to release OH ions which also neutralise the acid.

$$Ca_3(PO_4)_2 \rightleftharpoons 3Ca^{++} + 2PO_4^{\equiv}$$
$$PO_4^{\equiv} + HCl \rightleftharpoons HPO_4^{=} + Cl^{-}$$
$$PO_4^{\equiv} + HOH \rightleftharpoons HPO_4^{=} + OH^{-}$$

Tribasic calcium phosphate is official in I.P.

Official Tests for Identity: Gives the reactions characteristic of calcium, and of phosphates (refer Chapter 13).

Standard: Contains not less than 34 per cent and not more than 40 per cent of calcium and not less than 90 per cent of calcium phosphate, calculated with reference to the ignited substance.

Storage Condition: Store in a well-closed container.

Chemical Incompatibility: Same as for calcium chloride.

Medicinal and Pharmaceutical Use: Pharmaceutical aid (excipient). Sometimes it is used as a **gastric antacid.**

CHAPTER 11
RADIO PHARMACEUTICALS AND CONTRAST MEDIA

I. ATOMIC STRUCTURE

Matter is made up of atoms. An atom is composed of a very small, very dense, positively charged nucleus surrounded by sufficient number of negatively charged electrons in different orbits so that the atom is electrically neutral. Practically all the mass of the atom is in the nucleus.

The nucleus contains positively charged protons and neutrons. The neutrons have no charge. The number of protons in the nucleus is known as the atomic number (Z). It is equal to the number of electrons revolving around the nucleus. The mass number (A) is the number of protons and neutrons in the nucleus. The mass number represents the weight of the atom (atomic weight),since the weight of the electrons is negligible.

The hydrogen atom is the lightest of the atomic species. It contains only one proton in the nucleus which is surrounded by one electron. The heaviest naturally occurring element is uranium. It contains in its nucleus 92 protons and 146 neutrons. To represent an atom with all the above details, its symbol is written as below:

$$_Z^A X \qquad \begin{aligned} &(A - \text{Mass number} \\ &Z - \text{Atomic number} \\ &X - \text{Symbol of element)} \end{aligned}$$

Examples:

1. Hydrogen $\quad _1^1H \qquad$ (M.N. = 1
$\qquad\qquad\qquad\qquad\quad$ A.N. = 1)

2. Lithium $\quad _3^7Li \qquad$ (M.N. = 7
$\qquad\qquad\qquad\qquad\quad$ A.N. = 3)

3. Nitrogen $\quad _7^{14}N \qquad$ (M.N. = 14
$\qquad\qquad\qquad\qquad\quad$ A.N. = 7)

4.	Oxygen	$^{16}_{8}O$	(M.N. = 16 A.N. = 8)
5.	Sodium	$^{23}_{11}Na$	(M.N. = 23 A.N. = 11)
6.	Chlorine	$^{35}_{17}Cl$	(M.N. = 35 A.N. = 17)

II. ISOTOPES

Sometimes an atom of an element (known as a nuclide) may have the same number of protons in the nucleus but the number of neutrons may be different. Therefore its mass number is different while the atomic number is the same. This is called an isotope of the element.

Isotopes occur in nature and an element may be considered to be a mixture of isotopes. However the isotopes occur mixed in the same proportions always. Thus the atomic weight is always the same because it is the average weight of all the atoms in the isotopic mixture.

Examples of Isotopes

1. Isotopes of hydrogen $^{1}_{1}H$, $^{2}_{1}H$ and $^{3}_{1}H$
   (Hydrogen, deuterium and tritium)

2. Isotopes of carbon $^{12}_{6}C$ and $^{13}_{6}C$

3. Isotopes of oxygen $^{16}_{8}O$, $^{17}_{8}O$ and $^{18}_{8}O$

4. Isotopes of Chlorine $^{35}_{17}Cl$, $^{37}_{17}Cl$ and $^{38}_{17}Cl$

5. Isotopes of iron $^{54}_{26}Fe$ and $^{56}_{26}Fe$

6. Isotopes of bromine $^{79}_{35}Br$ and $^{81}_{35}Br$

All the isotopes of an element follow the same chemical reactions. Therefore isotopes are chemically identical.

III. RADIOACTIVITY

The atoms of heavy elements such as uranium are unstable. In their nucleus the neutron to proton ratio is high. Only nuclei which have

142

almost the same number of neutrons and protons are stable. So the nucleus of elements like uranium-235 throw out or emit some particles such as the alpha particles or beta particles and also give out some radiation like the x-rays in order to attain stability. This is known as radioactivity.

Types of Radiations: The radiations emitted due to radioactivity are of three types. They can be easily separated by passing them between oppositely charged plates.

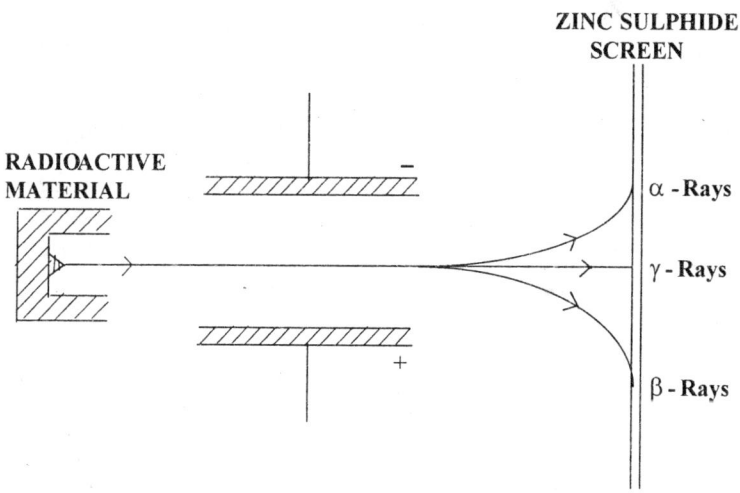

Figure

The radiation which bends towards the negatively charged plate must itself be positively charged and is known as alpha rays. That which bends towards the positively charged plate is obviously negatively charged itself and is known as beta rays. The third one which does not bend towards either the positively charged plate or the negatively charged plate but passes straight through is uncharged and is known as gamma rays.

Alpha Rays: Alpha rays consist of streams of alpha particles. They have two positive charges and a mass of 4 amu (atomic mass units). So they are helium nuclei and may be represented as $_2^4\alpha$ or $_2^4\text{He}$.

143

They have very high velocity equal to about one-tenth (1/10) of that of light. However their penetrating power through matter is very low. They can be stopped even by a sheet of paper. They have the capacity to cause intense ionisation in the molecules of gases through which they pass. This means that alpha rays, because of their positive charge and relatively high velocity, break off electrons in the gas molecules and produce ion-pairs (that is, electrons and positively charged ions).

Beta rays: Beta rays consist of streams of electrons. They have very small mass and a negative charge of one. A beta particle may be represented as $_{-1}^{0}\beta$ or $_{-1}^{0}e$. They move with a velocity equal to that of light. They are very much more penetrating than alpha rays. They can be stopped only by a 1 cm thick aluminium sheet. This is because of their small mass.

Gamma rays: Gamma rays do not consist of particles. They are radiation of wave form shorter than x-rays. They are usually emitted along with alpha rays or beta rays. They have neither mass nor charge and may be represented as $_{0}^{0}\gamma$. Gamma rays also move with the velocity of light and have the highest penetrating power. They can be stopped only by a 5 cm thick sheet of lead or concrete of many metres thickness. However they are very weak ionisers.

DETECTION AND MEASUREMENT OF RADIO ACTIVITY

There are several methods for detecting and measuring radioactive radiation. These are:

    1. Cloud chamber method.

    2. Ionisation chamber method.

    3. Geiger-Muller counter method.

    4. Scintillation counter method.

For our purpose the last two are important.

GEIGER-MULLER COUNTER

This consists of a cylindrical metal tube serving as the cathode and a central wire inside the tube serving as the anode (See figure). Argon gas is filled in the tube at a reduced pressure of 0.1 atmosphere.

$$A \rightarrow Ar^+ + e^-$$

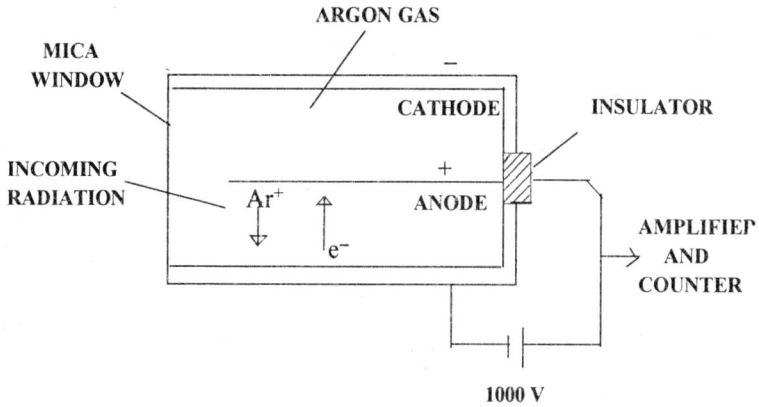

Figure

A potential difference of about 1000 volts is applied across the two electrodes. The argon gas is ionised whenever any alpha or beta particle enters the tube through the mica window. The positively charged argon ions, formed due to the ionisation of the gas, are attracted to the cathode and the negatively charged electrons to the anode. Thus an electrical pulse flows between the electrodes whenever one alpha or beta particle enters the tube. The electrical pulses are counted in an automatic counter. The intensity of the radioactivity of any radioactive material can be found out by finding the number of pulses per minute.

SCINTILLATION COUNTER

Scintillation means a flash of light. In this counter the radioactive substance mounted on a wire emits alpha particles. Each alpha particle strikes a zinc sulphide screen and gives a flash. The flashes produced per second can be counted to find out the intensity of radiation.

In the well-type scintillation counter, instead of the zinc sulphide screen a crystal of sodium iodide mixed with a little thallium iodide is used. The sample of the radioactive substance is kept in a well cut in the crystal. The radiation from the radioactive substance strikes the crystal wall and produces flashes. These scintillations fall on a photoelectric cell which converts the light energy into electrical energy for each flash. These are counted in a counter, even upto one million scintillations per second. This counter can be used for counting either alpha or beta particles.

IV. BIOLOGICAL EFFECTS OF RADIATION

Humans may at times be exposed to radiation from various sources such as cosmic rays, x-rays (in diagnostic procedures), monazite sands of Kerala containing radioactive thorium etc. Abnormally we may be exposed to the intense radiation due to the testing and explosion (as in Hiroshima and Nagasaki in 1945) of fission bombs (atom bombs) and radiation due to leakage from nuclear reactors such as the Chernobyl nuclear disaster in Russia in which the radiation was carried to many parts of Europe from Russia as a fallout.

Therefore in this context there is need to study the biological effects of radiation. The radiations that can produce damage are alpha particles, beta particles, protons, neutrons, gamma rays and x-rays. They do so by ionization and excitement of molecules in cells. One theory says that they ionize the water present in the cells to the extent of 80% and produce free radicals. These free radicals are highly unstable and very active. They react with each other and also with organic molecules in the cells producing a variety of secondary chemical substances such as peroxides which are very injurious to the cell. The DNA in the cell is particularly sensitive and is damaged, destroying the cell. There is also inhibition of mitosis or cell division.

The damage caused by radiation may be divided into two types.

1. Somatic effects, affecting the various parts of the body.

2. Genetic efects, affecting the reproduction and heredity.

The initial symptoms in humans are severe nausea, vomiting and prostration. After a few hours diarrhoea comes on due to ulceration of the gut with bleeding. Red cells, lymphocytes, blood platelets and granulocytes are found to be reduced in number, leading to anaemia etc. Antibody production is decreased and the body resistance comes down promoting infection. Death will follow after 2 to 3 weeks after a heavy dose of radiation.

Delayed Effect of Radiation

Continuous exposure to low level radiation can give rise to delayed effects of radiation. The hair greys quickly and other degeneraive changes take place leading to premature ageing. Several types of cancer are induced. These include cancer of skin, lung cancer, leukemia, Hodgkin's disease etc. Large doses of radiation may inactivate the gonads leading to sterility. Radiation exposure also produces chromosomal damage giving rise to mutations and consequent decreased fertility.

V. ARTIFICIAL RADIO ACTIVITY

Artificial radio activity can be brought about by bombarding a suitable element with neutrons (slow neutrons are very effective). This disturbs the nucleus which becomes unstable. To regain stability it starts disintegrating and emitting some rays and thus has become radioactive.

The radio active isotopes of certain elements have been used as tracers in various types of investigations. The stable element and a little of its radioactive isotope are mixed and converted to the required compounds. The compounds are now said to be labelled. The stable and the radioactive isotopes go through all physical and chemical changes in the same ratio. Thus the compound can be estimated by simply measuring the radioactivity of the active isotope. Biochemical and physiological properties of certain compounds can be studied like this. For this a mixture of stable and radioisotopes is fed to an animal. It may be distrubuted to different parts of the body or concentrated in one particular part of the body. Thus sodium radioiodide is absorbed mainly by the thyroid gland.

Important artificial radio nuclides used in medicine are cobalt-60 (used, like radium, for the treatement of cancer), phosphorus-32 (used in blood studies) and iodine-131 (used in the diagnosis and treatment of thyroid disease).

VI. MEDICAL USES OF RADIO ISOTOPES

1. Radiation Sterilization: Thermo-labile drugs such as penicillin may be sterilized by radiation from radio nuclides. All microorganisms and their spores are killed within seconds and the drug becomes sterile. Gamma rays from radio-isotopes are used for this purpose in addition to high speed electrons.

2. Radio Therapy: Here the aim is to destroy diseased tissue without destroying healthy tissue.Gamma radiation, being the most penetrating, is used for destroying deep-seated tumours. Both external and internal therapy are used. X-radiation can only be used for external therapy. In internal therapy the radio nuclide is placed in a natural or surgical cavity of the body or injected into the tissue. Sometime, there is selective uptake by a diseased organ. Gamma-emitter iodine-131 is given orally and is taken up by the thyroid. Sources with a short half-life such as iodine-131 and gold-198 can be left in the body permanently but sources such as radium-226 with a long half-life must be removed after the treatment is over.

3. Radio Diagnosis: Many materials which are opaque to visible light are tranparent to x-rays and gamma rays.

The function of a particular organ may be studied by following or tracing the manner in which it secretes or removes a particular radio-isotope eg. iodine (given in the form of sodium radioiodide) is taken up by the thyroid gland. This can be easily followed by a radiation detector. Another use of iodine-131 is in the form of diiodofluorescein used to map out a brain tumour before surgery.

Storage of Radio Isotopes: It is necessary to protect people from the harmful radiations emitted by the radioisotopes since we earlier studied about the harmful biological effects caused by the radiations. For this purpose the radioisotopes should be kept in remote places in the general store where people should not be allowed to go. The radioisotopes emitting gamma rays should be kept in lead containers of suitable thickness, as gamma rays are most penetrating. Alpha and beta ray emitters should be kept in thick glass containers, as alpha and beta rays are not as penetrating as gamma rays. The area where the radioactive materials are kept should be monitored regularly for radioactivity and any untoward increase in radiation should be detected in time and remedial measures taken.

Precautions in the Use of Radioisotopes: The following precautions should be observed while handling the radio isotopes:

1. Glass apparatus and other equipment should be tested for radioactivity before use.

2. Rubber gloves should be used while handling radioactive materials.

3. Absorbent paper should be used while handling radioactive liquids so that any liquid spilled may be absorbed by the paper and the paper thrown out.

4. Pipettes should not be used for withdrawing or tranferring radioactive liquids.

Half-life Period: The rate of disintegration of a radio active element is independent of temperature, pressure or its state of chemical combination. The time required for the disappearance of one half of the original amount of the radio active substance is called its Half–life Period.

VII. UNITS OF RADIO ACTIVITY

The unit of radio activity is the Curie (Ci). It is the weight of any radio active substance undergoing the same number of distintegrations per second as 1 g of radium, which is 3.7×10^{10} disintegrations per second. Each disintegration is also known as a becquerel (Bq) . Therefore 1 curie is equal to 3.7×10^{10} becquerels. Curie is a large unit; so in its place smaller units such as millicuries and microcuries are used frequently. One millicurie is one-thousandth ($\frac{1}{1000}$) of a curie and therefore represents 3.7×10^{7} disintegrations per second or becquerels. Likewise one microcurie is one–thousandth ($\frac{1}{1000}$) of a millicurie and so represents 3.7×10^{4} disintegrations per second or becquerels. It is stressed that the weight of any radioactive substance with a radioactivity of one curie need not be 1 g as in the case of radium but may be different.

VIII. RADIO PHARMACEUTICALS IN MEDICAL PRACTICE

The following are some of the radio pharamaceuticals official in B.P. 1988.

1. FERRIC CITRATE (^{59}Fe) INJECTION

This is a sterile solution containing (^{59}Fe) iron in the ferric state. It also contains 1 per cent of sodium citrate and also enough sodium chloride to make the solution isotonic with blood serum. Neutron irradiation of iron-58 produces the radio-active isotope, iron-59. Its half-life is 44.6 days only. The iron-58 selected for radiation should be sufficiently low in the content of iron-54. Otherwise the radioactive isotope, iron-55 may also be produced. Since it has a half-life of 2.87 years, its presence in this injection is not desirable. Therefore a limit of 2 per cent is prescribed on the content of iron-55 in the total activity. Hence before the iron-58 is irradiated to get radioactive iron-59, any iron-54 present along with iron-58 is electromagnetically separated so that the product will be able to comply with this provision of the content of iron-55 not to exceed 2 per cent of total activity. Radioactive isotope ^{59}Fe is capable of emitting both beta particles and gamma rays. It is sterilised by Heating in an Autoclave. The following are the official standards that the injection is required to comply with:

Description: A clear, colourless or faintly orange-brown solution.

Tests for Identity

(a) It has already been indicated that it emits gamma rays. Therefore the gamma ray spectrum of the injection should be compared with the gamma ray spectrum of an already standardised iron-59 solution. The two must be identical. Further the principal energies of the gamma rays should be 1.10 and 1.29 MeV (million electron volts). The activity of the injection also decays with a half-life of 44.6 days.

(b) When the injection is boiled with mercuric sulphate solution and potassium permanganate is added, the potassium permanganate is decolourised and a white precipitate is produced. This is a general test for citrates.

pH: 6 to 8

Radionuclidic Purity: The gamma ray spectrum of the injection is compared with the gamma ray spectrum of a standardised iron-59 solution. There should be no significant difference indicating that the injection contains only the required iron-59 isotope. In short this is a test for isotopic purity (refer also the first Test for Identity). If any iron-55 is present it may not be detected by this test.

Total Iron: The amount of iron present is limited by this test. In this test a volume of the substance equivalent to 10 microcuries is subjected to the limit test for iron and required to comply with it.

Sterility: Since this a parenteral preparation, it must comply with the test for sterility. However the B.P. states that the preparation may be released for use before completion of the test. Because of the radioactive nature of the preparation, it is not always possible to wait for final results of the test for sterility for use of the batch.

Standard: The content of iron-59 should be between 90 and 110 per cent of what is stated on the label on the particular date stated on the label. The specific activity is not less than 1 microcurie per mg of iron (37 megabecquerels) on the date stated on the label.

Assay: It is assayed for its activity by detection of its gamma radiation in a scintillation counter and comparing it with the activity of a standardised iron-59 solution.

Use: In the investigation of blood disorders.

2. SODIUM IODIDE (^{131}I) SOLUTION

This solution is suitable for oral administration and it contains iodine-131 in the form of sodiun iodide. Sodium thiosulphate or other suitable reducing agent is also preent. By irradiating tellurium with neutrons, we can obtain the radioactive isotope of iodine, iodine-131 which is converted to sodium radioiodide.

Description: It is a clear, colourless solution. It has a half-life of 8.06 days and emits both beta particles and gamma rays.

Test for Identity: The gamma ray spectrum of this solution is compared with the gamma ray spectrum of a standardised iodine-131 solution. There should be no significant difference. Further the principal gamma-photon has an energy of 0.36 MeV.

151

pH: 7 to 10.

Radionuclidic purity: The gamma ray spectrum measured in a suitable instrument is compared with the gamma ray spectrum of a standardised iodine-131 solution. There should be no significant difference.

This test is meant to ensure the absence of isotopes other than sodium (^{131}I) iodide.

Radiochemical purity: This test is meant to ensure that all the radioactivity is present only in the iodide ion and not because of the presence of some other iodine-containing compound such as the iodate.

It is done by paper chromatography. In this it should be proved 'that the radioactive part of the paper chromatogram coincides with the position of the iodide ion. It should also be proved that the position corresponding to the iodate ion has no radioactivity.

Standard: The content of iodine-131 actvity should be between 90 and 100 per cent of that stated on the label at the time and hour stated on the label. The specific activity is not less than 5 mCi per microgram or 185 MBq (megabecquerals) per microgram of iodine at the date and hour stated on the label.

Assay: By using a suitable counter, the activity is compared with the activity of a standardised iodine-131 solution. It should have the iodine-131 activity and specific activity as prescribed.

Use: Used for the diagnosis and treatment of disorders of the thyroid gland.

3. SODIUM PHOSPHATE (^{32}P) INJECTION

This is a sterile solution of disodium and monosodium orthophosphates in isotonic saline. Phosphorus-32 is produced by the neutron irradiation of sulphur and is a radioactive isotope of phosphorus. It emits only beta particles with an energy of 1.71 MeV. It has a half-life of 14.3 days. The injection should comply with the general requirements for all injections and in addition should comply with the following also:

Description: A clear, colourless solution.

Tests for Identity: The beta ray spectrum or the beta ray absorption curve of the injection is measured and compared with that of a phosphorus-32 solution obtained under the same conditions. There should be no significant difference. The beta radiation has also an energy of 1.7 MeV.

pH: between 6 and 8.

Radionuclidic Purity: This is to prove that the radio activity in the solution comes only from the radioisotope phosphorous-32 and not from any other radioisotope. For this purpose the beta-ray spectrum or the beta-ray absorption curve is measured and compared with that of a standardised phosphorus-32 solution obtained under the same conditions. There should be no significant difference.

Radiochemical Purity: This test is designed to prove that all the radioactivity resides in the phosphate ion and not in any other ion such as the phosphite. For this purpose the solution is first diluted to an activity of about 20,000 counts per minute. This dilution is then subjected to paper chromatography separately along with inactive orthophosphoric acid. The position of the inactive phosphoric acid is determined by spraying perchloric acid and ammonium molybdate solutions and then exposing to hydrogen sulphide when a blue colour develops. The radioactive spot is then located by using a suitable instrument and measured. Not less than 95 per cent of the total radioactivity should be present in the spot corresponding to the orthophosphoric acid.

Total Phosphate: The amount of phosphate is limited by diluting the solution with water and treating with ammonium metavanadate, ammonium molybdate and perchloric acid solutions. The colour produced after diluting to the specified volume is compared with the colour produced in a standard solution prepared at the same time and under the same conditions and containing a definite amount of orthophosphate. The colour in the test solution should not be more intense than the colour in the standard solution.

Sterility: The test for sterility is done. However the preparation may be released for use before the completion of the test.

Standard: The content of phosphorus-32 activity is between 90 and 110 percent of that stated on the label at the date and hour stated on the label. The specific activity is not less than 0.3 mCi (11.1MBq) per mg of orthophosphate ion.

Assay: The activity is determined by comparing with a standardised phosphorus-32 solution by using a suitable instrument.

Use: Used in the treatment of polycythaemia vera.

IX. X-RAY CONTRAST MEDIA

Most of the body tissues are transparent to x-rays which means x-rays are able to pass through them. However some chemicals such as barium sulphate are opaque to x-rays, that is they block the passage of x- rays. These substances are known as radio-opaque media or x-ray contrast media. They are used for diagnostic purposes. For example in the case of barium sulphate, it is made into a suspension with water and administered either orally or rectally by injection. The barium sulphate coats the mucosa of the gut and when x-rays are allowed to pass through and fall on an x-ray film, diseases such as ulcers etc, are mapped out.

BARIUM SULPHATE, BaSO$_4$

Preparation: It is prepared by treating a cold, dilute solution of any soluble barium salt such as barium chloride with dilute sulphuric acid.

$$BaCl_2 + H_2SO_4 \longrightarrow BaSO_4\downarrow + 2HCl$$

The preciptate is filtered with water, washed and dried.

Physical and Chemical Properties

Barium sulphate is a fine, heavy, white powder, free from gritty particles. It is odourless and tasteless. It is insoluble in water and organic solvents and also in dilute acids and alkalis. It is soluble in concentrated sulphuric acid.

Since barium sulphate is practically insoluble, it is not very reactive chemically. However it can be fused with one or both of the alkali carbonates such as sodium carbonate and potassium carbonate.

$$BaSO_4 + Na_2CO_3 \longrightarrow Na_2SO_4 + BaCO_3$$

The barium carbonate may be neutralised by any acid to yield a soluble barium salt and the mixture now answers tests for barium. The filtrate after removal of the barium carbonate in the above reaction also answers the reactions of sulphate.

It is official in I.P.

Official Tests for Identity

1. A small quantity of the sample is boiled with sod.carbonate solution, filtered and the filtrate acidified with dilute hydrochloric acid. It now answers the reactions of sulphates (see Chapter 13).

2. The residue obtained in (1) above is washed with water and treated with dilute hydrochloric acid. It is filtered and dilute sulphuric acid is added. A white preciptate is formed and it is insoluble in dilute hydrochloric acid (refer physical and chemical properties).

Standard: Barium sulphate contains between 97.5 per cent and 100.5 per cent of $BaSO_4$.

Storage Condition: Since barium sulphate is very stable, it is enough if it is stored in well-closed containers.

Chemical Incompatibility: Since barium sulphate is practically insoluble and also since it is not dispensed in solution, the question of chemical incompatibility is ruled out.

Medicinal and Pharmaceutical Use: Diagnostic aid (radio–opaque medium). It is used in the form of a suspension or rarely as a rectal injection.

Caution: I.P. prescribes tests for sulphide and soluble barium salts which are very poisonous. Therefore if these salts are present, such a sample of barium sulphate should not be used as it will kill the patient.

CHAPTER 12

QUALITY CONTROL OF DRUGS AND PHARMACEUTICALS

I. IMPORTANCE OF QUALITY CONTROL

The drugs and pharmaceuticals used in the prevention and treatment of diseases are derived from plant, animal or mineral origin or made synthetically. Usually they are not available in a state of purity since many other substances known as impurities are also present along with them. Therefore it is necessary not only to identify these impurities but also to precisely estimate their amount so that we can decide whether they are within the permitted limits. Similarly the drug should be present in the sample in the quantity prescribed for effective action. This can be ascertained by estimation of the drug constituent. Unless we find out that a drug complies with all the standards prescribed, we will be in the dark about not only its efficacy but also its stability, safety and purity. So the quality control of drugs and pharmaceutical formulations is very important and enables us to achieve this objective.

II. ERRORS IN QUALITY CONTROL

In any analysis errors may be present to make the results obtained in the analysis unreliable. Therefore it is necessary to have full knowledge of the sources of these errors so that they may be eliminated or reduced ensuring that the results of the analysis will be reliable. The errors are of two types:

1. Indeterminate or accidental errors.

2. Determinate or constant errors.

Indeterminate errors are not easily observable and their elimination also is impossible, since indeterminate errors are caused by differences in judgement and also skill of the analysts. It means that two analysts analysing the sample of a drug may not get identical results, if they do not have the same skill in performing the analysis and also if their awareness of the intricacies of the analysis is different.

Determinate errors are those which occur again and again in a series of determinations in the analysis of a drug. These errors may be caused because the analyst commits some errors unwittingly such as that he is not taking a representative sample of the drug or that his selection of the indicator for the analysis is wrong or that he overshoots the end point since he is unable to judge the colour change of the indicator at the end point properly. If the apparatus used in the analysis auch as pipetes and burettes are not properly calibrated or if the balance used for weighing the drug suffers from some defect such as inequality in the length of the arms or if incorrect weights are used, it will also contribute to the determinate errors. However these errors can be easily identified and rectified if proper care is taken.

Significant errors: In the number 145, the digits 1,4 and 5 are known as significant numbers. In the number 10.6, the zero is also a significant figure. In the number 1.000, all the zeros are significant figures. In the number 10.6, the zero lies to the left of the decimal and together with the other numbers gives the value of the number. In the other example, the zeros lie to the right of the decimal. Though normally they do not seem to have any value because 1.000 is equal to 1 only, yet if it is considered to be the weight of a substance, it means that the weight has been determined to an accuracy of 1 mg. In this sense the zeros are considered to be significant figures.

In an analysis all measurements can be carried out only with a certain amount of accuracy which means that some error is always there. For example let us assume that we are doing a titration using a burette calibrated to 0.01 ml. The titre value obtained is 22.5 ml. It means that the correct titre value lies somewhere between 22.45 and 22.55 ml. Therefore it is better to do a series of titrations and obtain the average of the titre values. Suppose five titrations are done and the titre values obtained are 22.45, 22.46, 22.48, 22.52 and 22.53 ml. The mean or average of these five titre values is 22.488. However if it is taken as 22.488, it would be a mistake of taking too many figures than necessary since it extends it to a third decimal, thereby indicating that the error of measurement is 0.0005 ml. So it should be rounded off to 22.49 and the error on account of this eliminated.

III. METHODS OF QUALITY CONTROL

As per the pharmacopoeia, the official drug or pharmaceutical formulation has to comply with the following standards:

1. **Description of the drug**: A brief description of the drug including odour and taste. Example: A white, crystalline solid with a bitter taste and a characteristic odour.

2. **Tests for Identity**: By doing these tests for identity, we can prove that the sample is nothing but the particular drug.

3. **Physical Constants**: Physical constants are the characteristic properties of the particular drugs. If the drugs comply with the physical constants, it means the drugs are pure. In addition, physical constants also serve as additional tests for identity. The following are the important physical constants, some of which may be prescribed for particular drugs:

   (a) **Melting Point**: If the drug melts sharply at the stated melting point, it means that the drug is pure. Additionally melting point is also a test for identity.

   (b) **Solubility**: Solubility in particular solvents serves as a test for identity.

   The other physical constants prescribed are -

   (c) **Weight per ml (for liquids) or specific gravity.**

   (d) **Refractive index.**

   (e) **Optical rotation.**

   (f) **Viscosity.**

   (g) **Light absorption in the visible and ultraviolet ranges.**

   (h) **Infrared absorption etc.**

4. **Limit tests**: Limit tests are done to ensure that impurities, if present in the drug, are within the permitted limits.

5. **Assay**: Assay is done to estimate precisely the amount of the drug in the sample or the active ingredients in any formulation. The following assay methods are used :-

   (a) Volumetric methods such as acid-base titrations, oxidation-reduction titrations, precipitation titrations, complexo-metric titrations, non-aqueous titrations etc.

(b) Gravimetric analysis in which a drug or a derivative of the drug is finally weighed.

(c) Instrumental methods of analysis such as colorimetry, spectrophotometry, flame photometry etc.

IV. IMPURITIES AND LIMIT TESTS

1. IMPURITIES IN PHARMACOPOEIAL SUBSTANCES

Chemical purity means freedom from all foreign materials. It is not possible to obtain an absolutely pure compound and even analytically pure samples contains minute traces of other substances which are called as impurities. Purification of chemicals is expensive and therefore purifying a substance to a much higher degree than is necessary for the purpose for which it is intended to be used will increase its cost too much.

However it is possible at a comparatively less cost to mass produce certain substances in a high state of purity. Refined sugar contains more than 99.9 per cent of sucrose. Similarly vacuum salt contains more than 99.9 per cent of sodium chloride. It is made by purifying rock salt.

The Different Types of impurities Commonly Occurring in Drugs

1. Impurities which are toxic and produce unpleasant reactions in the body when present beyond certain limits, e.g. lead and arsenic.

2. Impurities which, though otherwise harmless, are present in such proportions that is not desirable. The presence of sodium bromide in the more expensive potassium bromide is not likely to cause harm to the patient. However medicinal quality potassium bromide should contain only potassium bromide and not contain large quantities of sodium bromide.

3. Impurities which bring down the keeping properties of the substances. For example a small amount of moisture may cause many substances to be easily oxidised or to undergo hydrolysis.

159

4. Impurities which render the medicament incompatible with other substances.

5. Impurities which cause what are known as technical difficulties in the use of the substance, for example presence of potassium iodate in a sample of potassium iodide. Such a sample will liberate iodine on being mixed with a mineral acid due to the interaction of both the substances.

6. Impurities which contribute a different odour or colour to the main substance and so are not desirable. Sodium salicyate is often discoloured due to phenolic impurities. Sodium chloride becomes damp due to the presence of traces of deliquescent magnesium salts.

Generally medical compounds should not only be free from undue amounts of toxic and undesirable substances but should also be of a reasonably pure quality. Those impurities, such as lead and arsenic which have deleterious effects, should not be present in amounts likely to be harmful. Very low limits are fixed for such impurities. Similarly very low limits are fixed for the other types of impurities also stated above for the reasons mentioned. However if the impurity is harmless and is at the same time difficult to remove, the limits may be fixed even as high as 5–10%.

Sources of Impurities in Pharmacopoeial Substances:

Impurities in pharmacopoeial substances may be due to the following sources:

(a) Raw materials used in manufacture

A good example is the presence of tin, lead, silver, copper, cobalt and gold in bismuth salts. These metals occur along with bismuth in bismuth ores. Rock salt contains small amounts of calcium and magnesium salts so that sodium chloride prepared from rock salt may contain traces of calcium and magnesium salts.

(b) The method of manufacture

Contamination by reagents and solvents at various stages of the manufacturing process may give rise to impurities as given below:

(i) *Reagents employed in the process.* Lead as an impurity may result from the sulphuric acid used as reagent, especially if it has been prepared by the lead chamber process. Soluble alkali may be an impuritiy in calcium carbonate if the calcium carbonate is made by reacting calcium chloride and sodium carbonate and not properly washed.

(ii) *Solvents.* Water is the solvent easily available and cheap and is used in the manufacture of inorganic chemicals. This can give rise to trace impurities such as sodium, calcium, magnesium, carbonate, chloride and sulphate ions. These difficulties do not arise in the use of purified water (distilled or demineralised water).

(iii) *The reaction vessels.* The vessels used in the manufacturing process are made of metals like copper, iron, aluminium, zinc, nickel and tin though these days many of these metals are replaced by stainless steel. The above metals are introduced as impurities due to the solvent action of the raw materials on the material of the plant. Glass vessels may give rise to traces of alkali, though this is unlikely if the vessels are made of neutral glass.

(c) Atmospheric contaminants

Atmospheric contamination may take place through dust, sulphur dioxide, hydrogen sulphide etc. Carbon dioxide and water vapour also contaminate substances which are affected by their action.

(d) Decomposition of the product during storage

Many chemical substances undergo changes due to careless storage. Ferrous sulphate is slowly changed into insoluble ferric oxide by air and moisture. Solution of potassium hydroxide absorbs carbon dioxide on exposure to air and exerts a solvent action on lead glass. Therefore it should be stored in well-stoppered bottles of green glass which is lead-free. There are certain precautions regarding storage and if they are observed, decomposition and deterioration of substances could be brought down if not totally eliminated. All chemicals should be stored in tightly closed containers made of dark glass and extremes of temperatures should be avoided. Sunlight affects many chemicals. For example bismuth carbonate turns black on exposure to sunlight for a long period. Such chemicals should be stored in a dark place preferably.

(e) Deliberate adulteration with spurious or useless materials

This is a still common occurrence iin some parts of the country where the Drugs and Cosmetics Act has not yet been properly enforced. Therefore one has to be vigilant and purchase drugs only from reputed manufacturers.

LIMIT TESTS

Limit tests are quantitative or semi-quantitative tests which are designed to detect and limit small quantities of impurities which are likely to be present in the substance. They may be of three types:

(a) Tests which show no visible reaction

It may be stated that on testing as prescribed there shall be no colour, opalescence or precipitate, whichever is relevant. Such negative tests only indicate the absence of an undesirably large amount of the impurity.

(b) Methods of Comparison

These tests need a standard containing a certain quantity of impurity and a test to be set up at the same time and under the same conditions. In this way, it is possible to compare the amount of the impurity in the substance with a standard of known concentration and find out whether the impurity is within or excess of the limit prescribed. This is the basis of the official limit tests for chloride, sulphate, iron etc.

(c) Quantitative Determinations

Here the amount of the impurity present is actually determined and compared with the numerical limit given in the pharmacopoeia.

Examples are:

1. Limits of soluble matter
2. Limits of insoluble matter
3. Limits of non-volatile matter

4. Limits of moisture and volatile matter
5. Limits of residue on ignition
6. Loss on ignition
7. Ash values

However we will limit out discussion to the comparison methods only. These limit tests involve simple comparisons of opalescence, turbidity or colour with the standards prescribed in the pharmacopoeias. The variations in the permissible limits for the various substances are obtained by taking varying quantities of the substance under test. In these limit tests the extent of opalescence, turbidity or colour produced is influenced by the presence of other impurities present in the substance and also by variations in time and method of performance of tests and hence the pharmacopoeias do not prescribe numerical values for these tests.

LIMIT TESTS FOR ACID RADICAL IMPURITIES

A. Limit Test for Chlorides (I.P.1985)

Principle: The limit test for chlorides is based on the well known reaction between silver nitrate and soluble chlorides forming a precipitate of silver chloride which is insoluble in dilute nitric acid. The test solution bcomes turbid, the extent of turbidity depending upon the amount of silver chloride produced which in turn depends upon the amount of chloride present in the test substance. The opalescence or turbidity so obtained is compared with the opalescence obtained in a standard solution containing a known quantity of chloride. The test is done in Nessler glasses, the same volume of dilute nitric acid is used in both the cases and both are diluted to the same volume. The standard turbidity is produced from the amount of chloride which is prescribed as the limit for chloride impurity in the test substance. If the turbidity from the sample is less than the standard turbidity, the sample passes the limit test. If it is more, it fails the limit test. The solutions must be viewed transversely against a dark background.

$$Cl^- + AgNO_3 \longrightarrow AgCl\downarrow + NO_3^-$$

Practical Details: A specified weight of the substance (accurately weighed) is dissolved in water or the solution is prepared by special treatment as given in the monograph in a Nessler cylinder. 10 ml of dilute nitric acid are added to the solution and the volume is made upto 50 ml with water (distilled or purified water only). 1 ml of silver nitrate is then added and the solution is stirred and set aside for 5 minutes.

Standard opalescence is likewise obtained by taking 1 ml of a 0.05845 per cent w/v solution of sodium chloride and 10 ml of dilute nitric acid in a Nessler cylinder, making upto 50 ml with water (distilled or purified water only) and adding 1 ml of silver nitrate solution. It is also stirred well and set aside for five minutes.

As already stated, when viewed transversely preferably against a dark background, the turbidity in the test solution should not be greater than the turbidity in the standard solution. Then only the sample passes the test. Otherwise it fails.

Certain points may be noted:

1. Certain substances have to be specially treated for a solution to be made which can be used in the test. The procedure for this is given in the individual monograph.

2. It must be stressed that the standard must be *accurately* prepared. Otherwise the test will not be reliable. Therefore it is necessary that *exactly 1 ml of exactly 0.05845 per cent w/v solution of sodium chloride* should be taken as the source for chloride.

3. The total quantity at the conclusion of the test in each Nessler cylinder is 51 ml and not 50 ml.

4. The standard opalescence is produced by 0.000355 g of chlorine in 50 ml:

$$\frac{0.05845 \times 35.45 \times 1}{58.45 \times 100} = 0.000355 \text{ g of chlorine}$$

Finally the amount of chlorine is 7 parts per million (7 p.p.m.) :

$$\frac{0.000355 \times 1,000,000}{50} = 7 \text{ p.p.m.}$$

B. Limit Test for Sulphates (I.P. 1985)

Principle: This is based on the reaction between barium chloride and soluble sulphate in the presence of dilute hydrochloric acid. A turbidity is produced by the precipitation of barium sulphate in a fine state of division. This is compared with the turbidity produced in a standard containing a known quantity of sulphate and similarly treated. The test substance passes the limit test if the turbidity in it is less than that in the standard. If the turbidity is found to be more, then it fails the test. The barium sulphate reagent used contains barium chloride, sulphate-free alcohol and a small amount of potassium sulphate. The addition of potassium sulphate increases the sensitivity of the test. The ionic concentration in the reagent is so adjusted that the solubility product of barium sulphate is exceeded. Barium sulphate present in the reagent in a small quantity acts as a seeding agent for precipitation of barium sulphate, if sulphate is present in the substance under test. Alcohol prevents supersaturation and a more uniform turbidity is formed.

$$SO_4^{--} + BaCl_2 \longrightarrow BaSO_4\downarrow + 2Cl^-$$

Practical Details: A specific quantity of the substance (accurately weighed) is dissolved in water or solution is prepared as directed in the monograph in a Nessler cylinder. 2 ml of dilute hydrochloric acid is then added and it is diluted to 45 ml with water. 5 ml of Barium Sulphate Regeant is added. The liquid is stirred well and set aside for five minutes for the turbidity to develop. The standard is obtained by taking 1 ml of a 0.1089 per cent w/v solution of potassium sulphate in a Nessler cylinder and mixing with 2 ml of dilute hydrochloric acid. It is diluted to 45 ml with water. Then Barium sulphate Reagent (5 ml) is added. It is stirred well and set aside for five minutes.

As already stated, when viewed transversely preferably against a dark background, the turbidity in the test should not be greater than the turbidity in the standard. Then only the sample passes the test. Otherwise it fails.

Certain points may be noted:

1. This is the same as in the case of Limit Test for Chlorides.

2. The standard must be *accurately* prepared. Otherwise the test will not be reliable. *Exactly 1 ml of exactly 0.1089 per cent w/v solution of potassium sulphate* should be taken as the source for sulphate.

3. The standard opalescence is produced by 0.0006 g of sulphate.

$$\frac{0.1089 \times 96 \times 1}{174 \times 100} = 0.0006 \text{ g of sulphate.}$$

Finally the amount of sulphate is 12 parts per million (p.p.m)

$$\frac{0.0006 \times 1,000,000}{50} = 12 \text{ p.p.m.}$$

LIMIT TESTS FOR BASIC RADICAL (OR METALLIC) IMPURITIES

A. Limit Test for Iron (I.P. 1985)

Principle: This depends upon the reaction of iron with thioglycollic acid in the presence of citric acid and ammonia when a pale pink to deep reddish purple colour is produced. Citric acid forms a complex with iron and prevents its precipitation by ammonia. The colour produced is due to the formation of ferrous compound with thioglycollic acid (which is a co-ordination compound). This is stable in the absence of air and fades when exposed to air due to oxidation. The original state of oxidation of iron is immaterial, as thioglycollic acid is a reducing agent and reduces ferric iron to ferrous. Only because of this advantage this test has been selected as the limit test, since other tests such as the ammonium thiocyante test give reaction with only one type of iron like the ferric. The thioglycollic acid test is also considered to be more sensitive. Ferrous thioglycollate is colourless in acid or neutral solution. The colour develops only in the presence of alkali. The reactions are given below:

$$2Fe^{+++} + 2CH_2 \text{ SH. COOH} \rightarrow$$

$$\begin{array}{l} 2Fe^{++} + \text{S. CH}_2\text{. COOH} \\ \text{Ferrous} \quad | \qquad\quad + 2H^+ \\ \text{iron} \quad\; \text{S. CH}_2\text{. COOH} \end{array}$$

Ferric Iron Thioglycollic acid

$$Fe^{++} + 2CH_2 \text{ SH. COOH} \rightarrow$$

Ferrous thioglycollate
(Coordination compound)

Practical Details

A solution of the specified quantity of test substance is prepared in a Nessler cylinder. 2 ml of a 20% solution of iron-free citric acid and 0.1 ml of thioglycollic acid are added. The solution is then mixed and made alkaline with iron-free ammonia solution, diluted to 50 ml with water, stirred well and allowed to stand for five minutes. The colour obtained is compared with the standard colour, prepared similarly in a Nessler cylinder by taking 2 ml of Standard Iron Solution and similarly treating it and making upto 50 ml with water. The intensity of the colour in the test solution should be less than that in the standard so that it may be declared to have passed the test. If it is more, it fails the test.

Certain points may be noted:

1. A colour and not a turbidity or opalescence develops.

2. The colour in the test and the standard should be compared immediately after the five minutes allowed for full development of the colour is over. If there is any delay, the colour fades due to oxidation and the test becomes unreliable.

B. Limit Test for Heavy Metals (I.P. 1985)

Principle: Many heavy metals, such as lead, iron, copper, nickel, cobalt, bismuth etc., may occur as impurities in official substances. So their quantity is limited by inclusion of a limit test for heavy metals. The test is based on the reaction between hydrogen sulphide and many heavy metals resulting in the formation of their sulphides which may have colours varying from dark brown to black. Since so many metals are sought to be tested for, fixing of a standard for comparison is difficult. However a standard solution containing a definite quantity of lead nitrate is chosen for the purpose. The quantity is stated as the heavy metals limit and is expressed as parts of lead (by weight) per million parts of the substance. The usual limit for heavy metals in I.P. is 20 p.p.m. The sulphides formed in the test are distributed in colloidal state and produce brownish solutions.

There are three methods prescribed in the I.P. depending upon the type of metals involved. Method A is used for substances, which give clear, colourless solutions, when the test solution is prepared as given in the individual monograph. Method B is used for substances which do not give clear, colourless solutions. It is also used for substances which interfere with the precipitation of the contaminating heavy metals as their sulphides. Method C is used for substances which give clear, colourless solutions when they are dissolved in sodium hydroxide solution. While the precipitation of the metallic sulphides is carried out in methods A and B under moderately acid conditions, it is done in method C under alkaline conditions. It is, therefore, obvious that optimum conditions are being provided for the metals to be precipitated as their sulphides.

Method A

Two solutions are prepared.

1. Standard Solution: 2 ml of standard lead solution are diluted with water in a 50 ml Nessler cylinder. The pH is adjusted to a value between 3 and 4 by the addition of either dilute acetic acid Sp or dilute ammonia solution Sp and the solution is diluted to 35 ml with water.

2. Test Solution: The specified quantity of the substance is made into a solution in a 50 ml Nessler cylinder as prescribed in the individual monograph. Then it is diluted with water to 25 ml and adjusted to a pH between 3 and 4 by the addition of either dilute acetic acid Sp or dilute ammonia solution Sp. The solution is then diluted to 35 ml with water.

Procedure: To both the solutions 10 ml of freshly prepared hydregen sulphide solution is added, mixed and diluted with water to 50 ml. They are allowed to stand for five minutes and viewed downwards over a white surface. The colour produced in the test solution should not be darker than the colour produced in the standard solution. Then only the sample passes the test. Otherwise it fails.

Method B

Two solutions are prepared as in Method A

1. Standard solution: It is prepared in the same way as in Method A.

2. Test solution: Since the substances coming under this category may contain a lot of organic matter, the sample is taken in a crucible and the organic matter is destroyed by addition of nitric and sulphuric acids and ignition at 500° to 600°C in a muffle furnace. Then the residue is digested with hydrochloric acid and extracted with hot water.

This extract contains the heavy metals present in the substance. It is transferred to a 50 ml Nessler cylinder and adjusted to a pH between 3 and 4 either by the addition of dilute acetic acid Sp or dilute ammonia solution Sp. Then it is diluted to 35 ml.

Procedure: It is the same as under Method A.

Method C

Two solutions are prepared as under Method A

1. Standard solution: 2 ml of standard lead solution and 5 ml of sodium hydroxide solution are taken in a 50 ml Nessler cylinder, diluted with water to 50 ml and mixed.

2. Test solution: The test solution is prepared as given in the individual monograph in a 50 ml Nessler cyclinder. 20 ml of water and 5 ml of sodium hydroxide solution are added. It is diluted to 50 ml and mixed.

Procedure: To both the solutions are added 5 drops of sodium sulphide solution. Each solution is mixed and allowed to stand for five minutes. When viewed downwards over a white surface, the colour produced in the test solution should not be darker then the colour produced in the standard solution.

All the reagents used in the tests should be free fom heavy metals which is indicated by the suffix Sp.

C. Quantitative Test for Lead

Lead is one of the most undesirable and dangerous impurities in medicinal substances. The primary sources of lead in chemicals are the sulphuric acid used in manufacture and the use of lead or leadlined apparatus. Lead may also be absorbed from lead glass. For ex. potassium carbonate kept in a badly stoppered bottle becomes moist and absorbs lead from the glass container and hence its lead content increases. The B.P. uses one method as the limit test and the I.P. another.

Quantitative Test for Lead in B.P.

The test depends upon the formation of brownish colouration when sodium sulphide is added to dilute solution of lead salts, the intensity of the colouration varying with the quantity of lead present. Traces of other metals, particularly copper and iron, interfere with the

169

test since they also yield dark precipitates or coloration with sodium sulphide (refer the heavy metals test). Addition of ammonia and potassium cyanide prevents their precipitation as sulphides. So under these conditions only lead alone is precipitated. By this test it is possible to find out not only whether the lead impurity present in the substance under test is within the prescribed limit but also the exact amount of the impurity.

The apparatus consists of two Nessler cyclinders, which should be made of clear lead-free glass with the 50 ml position clearly marked. The special reagents used are labelled PbT. With the exception of the standard lead solution, the reagents must be lead-free.

Two standard solutions of the substance are prepared.

1. a primary solution containing a definite quantity of the substance.

2. an auxiliary solution containing a definte but much smaller quantity of the substance.

To the auxiliary solution only a definite volume of a standard very dilute solution of lead nitrate is added. To both the solutions are added excess of ammonia and potasium cyanide. Any difference in colour between both solutions should be adjusted by adding dilute solution of burnt sugar. The two solutions are diluted to 50 ml. Then sodium sulphide is added to both the solutions and stirred. The colour developed in the primary should be less than the colour developed in the auxiliary. Then only the substance contains lead within the limit.

Limit Test for Lead in I.P. (I.P. 1985)

This is known as the Diphenylthiocarbazone Test.

Diphenylthiocarbarzone or dithizone dissolves in choloroform and the solution is green in colour. It has the ability to extract lead as a complex from substances containing lead as impurity, if the substance is dissolved in water and made alkaline.

The solution of the sample is prepared as directed in the monograph and transferred to a separator. Some of the metals other than lead particularly iron are complexed by the addition of ammonium citrate solution Sp and hydroxylamine hydrochloride solution Sp. The solution is then made just alkaline by the addition of strong ammonia

170

solution. Other metals are kept complexed by the addition of potassium cyanide.

This solution is then extracted with dithizone in chloroform repeatedly. Lead dithizonate is red in colour and the resultant colour (along with the green colour of unchanged dithizone) is a shade violet. Extraction is continued till the dithizone extraction solution remains green. This indicates that all lead has been extracted.

Nitric acid is added to the combined extract which converts all the lead dithizonate into lead nitrate. It is again extracted with dithizone extraction solution in the presence of ammonium cyanide. The colour of the extract is not a deeper shade of violet than that of a standard solution made with required quantity of lead solution similarly treated.

The double extraction is intended to ensure that only lead is extracted and all other metals are excluded. All reagents used with the exception of dilute standard lead solution should be lead free and are marked as Sp.

C_6H_5—N=NCS—NH—NH—C_6H_5
Dithizone

Dithizone-Lead Complex

D. Limit Test for Arsenic (I.P.1985)

Principle: The substance (which is supposed to contain the arsenic impurity) is dissolved in hydrochloric acid or an aqueous solution or extract is acidified. The arsenic present in the substance is converted to either arsenious acid (if the arsenic is trivalent) or arsenic acid (if the arsenic is pentavalent). Then it is further treated with a reducing agent such as stannous chloride or sulphurous acid. In the I.P. stannated hydrochloric acid (i.e.stannous chloride mixed with hydrochloric acid) is added to the substance.

$$H_3ASO_4 \longrightarrow H_3AsO_3$$
Arsenic acid   Arsenious acid

The arsenious acid is further reduced to arsine (arsenious hydride, AsH_3) by nascent hydrogen which is produced by the action of granulated zinc and hydrochloric acid.

$$H_3AsO_3 + 6H_2 \longrightarrow AsH_3 + 3H_2O$$
Arsine

When arsine comes into contact with dry paper saturated with mercuric chloride, it produces a yellow or brown stain.

$$2AsH_3 + HgCl_2 \longrightarrow Hg\,(AsH_2)_2 + 2HCl$$
Yellow or brown stain

The intensity of the stain is compared by daylight with a standard stain which is similarly prepared but taking a specified quantity of standard dilute arsenic solution in place of the substance. If the test stain is less in intensity than the standard stain, the sample passes the test. Otherwise it fails. This test is a modified Gutzeit test.

Practical Details:

A. Apparatus: The apparatus consists of a wide-mouthed glass bottle fitted with a rubber bung. A glass tube of specified dimensions is passed through the rubber bung. The internal diameter of the tube (6.5 mm) is important and should be uniform throughout. The tube is open at the upper end but tapers to a small diameter at the lower end. Near the lower end a hole is present at the side to allow any condensed moisture to escape.

The tube is first lightly packed with cotton wool saturated with lead acetate and dried. This is to trap any hydrogen sulphide which may be formed during the reaction if any sulphur impurity is present in the substance. If this is not done, the hydrogen sulphide will affect the mercuric chloride paper.

The mercuric chloride paper is fixed at the upper end of the tube between two rubber bungs by means of a spring clip. The two rubber bungs contain the tube in two parts and the mercuric chloride paper is correctly positioned between them. All the reagents are designated as AsT. Except Dilute Arsenic Solution they should be arsenic–free (see figure).

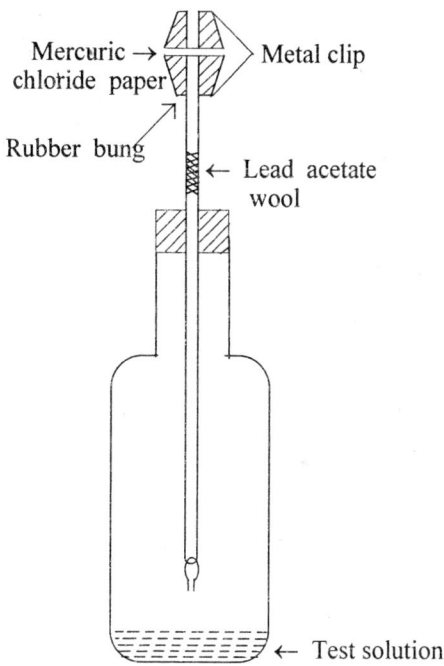

Mercuric → chloride paper

Metal clip

Rubber bung

← Lead acetate wool

← Test solution

Apparatus for Limit Test for Arsenic

B. Procedure: The solution of the substance to be examined is prepared as given in the monograph. Potassium iodide and arsenic-free zinc are added and the bottle is closed immediately with the cork carrying the attachments. The reaction is allowed to go on for forty minutes. A standard is also simultaneously done taking dilute solution of arsenic (specified quanity) in place of the substance and treating it similarly. The mercuric chloride paper in the test is removed and compared by daylight with the standard stain. The standard stains fade on keeping and should be freshly prepared.

CHAPTER 13

OFFICIAL IDENTIFICATION TESTS FOR ANIONS AND CATIONS

Identification tests are given in the I.P. 1985 for identifying the cations and anions of the inorganic substances included in the I.P. in monographs. Even though it is stated that these tests are not necessarily sufficient to establish absolute proof of identity, yet we can be reasonbly sure that the substance being tested is nothing but the substance claimed on the label, if it answers these tests for identification. When there is a doubt, there tests are hightly useful for establishing identity. Though the syllabus does not include all the inorganic substances official in the I.P., the tests for all the anions and cations given in the I.P. are included here to give a comprehensive idea to the student.

Anions are negatively charged ions or radicals which are attracted to the positively charged anode, while cations are positively charged ions attracted to the negatively charged cathode.

IDENTIFICATION TESTS FOR ANIONS

ACETATES

1. The sample is heated with an equal quantity of oxalic acid. Acetic acid with its characteristic odour is liberated.

2. The sample is heated with a little concentrated sulphuric acid and ethyl alcohol. The ester ethyl acetate,which can be recognised by its odour, is evolved.

3. To an aqueous solution of the sample are added successively lanthanum nitrate solution, decinormal iodine and dilute ammonia solution. The mixture is heated carefully to boiling. After a few minutes either a blue precipitate is formed or a dark blue colour develops.

4. If the substance is heated with a little calcium oxide, acetone is evolved. The acetone may be detected by the indigo blue colour it produces when its vapours are made to fall on a filter

paper moistened with a dilute solution of 2-nitro-benzaldehyde in alcohol, dried and further moistened with a 1N sodium hydroxide solution.

BENZOATES

1. To a neutral, aqueous solution of the sample is added a little Ferric Chloride T.S. A dull yellow precipitate, which is soluble in solvent ether, is formed.

2. A little of the sample is moistened with a little concentrated sulphuric acid in a test tube. When the bottom of the tube is gently warmed, no charring takes place. A white sublimate is deposited on the inner walls of the tube.

3. An aqueous solution of the sample is treated with a little concentrated hydrochloric acid. A precipitate is obtained. It is crystallised from water and dried under reduced pressure. It melts at about 122°C.

BICARBONATES AND CARBONATES

1. Solutions of bicarbonates, on boiling, liberate carbon dioxide which turns lime water milky. Carbonates do not give this reaction.

2. Solutions of bicarbonates give no precipitate with magnesium sulphate solutions but on boiling a white precipitate is produced. Solutions of carbonates give with magnesium sulphate solution a white precipitate at room temperature. The white precipitate is magnesium carbonate.

   In the test for bicarbonates, the soluble magnesium bicarbonate first formed decomposes on boiling to magnesium carbonate.

3. Aqueous solutions of carbonates and bicarbonates liberate carbon dioxide on being heated gently with dilute acetic acid. The gas is passed though barium hydroxide solution. A white precipitate of barium carbonate is formed. It dissolves on adding an excess of dilute hydrochloric acid.

BROMIDES

1. An aqueous solution of the sample is treated with a little dilute nitric acid and a little silver nitrate solution. A curdy pale yellow precipitate is formed. It is slightly soluble in dilute ammonia.

2. An aqueous solution of the sample is treated with chlorine solution. Bromine is evolved. The bromine solution is divided into two parts. To one part add 2 or 3 drops of chloroform. A reddish solution is formed in the chloroform layer. To the other part phenol solution is added. A white precipitate (of tribromophenol) is formed.

CARBONATES: Refer under Bicarbonates

CHLORIDES

1. Solutions of chlorides give with dilute nitric acid and silver nitrate solution a curdy, white precipitate of silver chloride. It is soluble in dilute ammonia solution but insoluble in dilute nitric acid.

2. A little of the sample in a test tube is mixed with a little potassium dichromate and a little concentrated sulphuric acid. A filter paper moistened with a dilute solution of diphenylcarbazide solution is placed over the opening of the test tube. The paper turns violet-red.

CITRATES

1. Neutral solutions of citrates, boiled with an excess of calcium chloride solution, give a white granular precipitate of calcium citrate. It is soluble in acetic acid.

2. An aqueous solution of the sample is mixed with acidified potassium permanganate solution and warmed till the colour of the permanganate is discharged. It is mixed with a little sodium nitroprusside solution in 2N sulphuric acid and sulphamic acid. It is made alkaline by adding strong ammonia solution drop by drop till the sulphamic acid is completely dissolved. Further addition of ammonia solution gives a violet colour changing to violet-blue.

IODIDES

1. Solutions of iodides give with dilute nitric acid and silver nitrate solution a curdy, yellow precipitate of silver iodide which is insoluble in dilute ammonia and in dilute nitric acid.

2. Iodides, when heated with sulphuric acid and potassium dichromate, produce violet coloured iodine. When a few ml of chloroform are added and shaken and allowed to settle, the chloroform layer is coloured violet or violet-red.

3. Solutions of iodides give with mercuric chloride solution a dark red precipitate (mercuric iodide). This is very soluble when excess of potassium iodide is added (potassium mercuric iodide is formed).

LACTATES

To an aqueous solution of the substance bromine water and dilute sulphuric acid are added and heated on a water bath till the colour is discharged. To this mixture ammonium sulphate and a solution of sodium nitroprusside in 2N sulphuric acid are added. Finally without mixing strong ammonia solution is added and allowed to stand for thirty minutes. A dark green ring appears at the place(interface) where the two liquids meet.

NITRATES

1. To an aqueous solution of the substance mixed with a little concentrated sulphuric acid is added ferrous sulphate solution through the sides of the test tube. A brown colour is formed at the interface of the two liquids.

2. A small quantity of the substance is added to a mixture of nitrobenzene and concentrated sulphuric acid. It is allowed to stand for five minutes and cooled in ice water while water and sodium hydroxide solution are added slowly with stirring. Then acetone is added, shaken and allowed to stand. The upper layer shows an intense violet colour.

NITRITES (I.P. '66)

1. Nitrites give off red fumes when heated with diluted sulphuric acid (nitrogen dioxide is liberated).

2. When dilute sulphuric acid, potassium iodide solution and starch solution are added to a solution of a nitrite, a blue colour is produced (potassium iodide is oxidised by the nitrous acid to iodine which gives the blue colour with starch).

3. A deep brown colour is produced when ferrous sulphate solution is added to a nitrite solution.

4. Solutions of nitrites, when treated with urea and dilute sulphuric acid, give off carbon dioxide which turns lime water milky.

PHOSPHATES

Solutions of orthophosphates give the following reactions:

1. Solution of an orthophosphate at pH 7 gives a light yellow precipitate with silver nitrate solution and dilute nitric acid.

2. Solution of an orthophosphate, when mixed with ammonia and magnesium sulphate solution, gives a white crystalline precipitate (magnesium ammonium phosphate).

3. Solution of an orthophosphate gives with dilute nitric acid and molybdate solution on warming a canary yellow precipitate (ammonium phosphomolybdate is produced).

SILICATES

Sodium fluoride and concentrated sulphuric acid are mixed with the sample in a platinum crucible to form a slurry. The crucible is covered with a thin, transparent plate of plastic. A drop of water is suspended from this plastic and gently warmed. A white ring is rapidly produced around the drop of water.

SALICYLATES

1. To a neutral solution of the substance Ferric Chloride T.S. is added. A violet colour is produced. The colour remains even after the addition of dilute acetic acid.

2. Concentrated hydrochloric acid is added to an aqueous solution of the substance. Salicylic acid is precipitated. It is recrystallised from hot water and dried in vacuum. It melts at about 159°C.

3. Bromine solution is added to a solution of the substance. A cream–coloured precipitate (of tribromosalicylic acid) is formed.

SULPHATES

1. Solutions of sulphates give with barium chloride solution a white precipitate (barium sulphate) which is insoluble in hydrochloric acid.

2. Solutions of sulphates give with solution of lead acetate a white precipitate (lead sulphate). It is soluble in ammonium acetate solution and also in sodium hydroxide solution.

3. To a suspension of barium sulphate in test (1) is added iodine solution. The suspension remains yellow but is decolourised by adding stannous chloride solution drop by drop. The mixture is boiled. No coloured precipitate is formed.

TARTRATES

1. Tartrates, when heated with concentrated sulphuric acid, char rapidly evolving carbon dioxide and carbon monoxide. The latter burns with a blue flame when ignited.

2. When a drop of ferrous sulphate solution is added to a solution of a tartrate acidified with acetic acid followed by a few drops of hydrogen peroxide, a transient yellow colour is produced. When sodium hydroxide solution is added drop by drop, a purple violet colour is produced.

3. Solutions of tartrates, mixed with potassium bromide solution and resorcinol solution and sulphuric acid, give an intense blue colour on warming cautiously. When the cooled solution is continuously poured into water, a red colour is obtained.

THIOSULPHATES

1. To an aqueous solution of the substance concentrated hydrochloric acid is added. A white precipitate which soon turns yellow (sulphur) is produced. Sulphur dioxide which can be recognised by its odour is evolved.

2. Ferric Chloride T.S. is added to a solution of the substance. A dark violet colour is produced and it quickly disappears.

3. Iodine solutions are decolourised by the addition of thiosulphate solutions. The decolourised solutions do not give the reactions of sulphates.

4. Bromine solution is decolourised by thiosulphate solution. The decolourised soltuion gives the reactions of sulphates.

IDENTIFICATION TESTS FOR CATIONS

AMMONIUM

1. Many ammonium salts volatilise on being heated strongly. No residue is left.

2. When ammonium salts are heated with sodium hydroxide solution, ammonia is produced. Ammonia can be easily recognised by its strong, pungent and characteristic odour. It turns moist red litmus paper blue. It also produces a black stain on a filter paper impregnated with mercurous nitrate.

ALUMINIU

1. To an aqueous solution of the substance, dilute hydrochloric acid and thioacetamide reagent are added. There is no precipitate. Dilute sodium hydroxide solution is added drop by drop. A gelatinous white precipitate is formed. More dilute sodium hydroxide solution is added. The precipitate is redissolved. Ammonium chloride solution is now added. The gelatinous white precipitate reappears.

2. A small quantity of ammonium acetate solution and a small quantity of mordant blue-3 solution are added to a solution of the substance. An intense purple colour is produced.

3. Dilute ammonia is added to an aqueous solution of the substance until a faint precipitate is produced. Then quinalizarin in sodium hydroxide solution is added. The mixture is heated to boiling, cooled and acidified with excess of acetic acid. A reddish -violet colour is produced.

ANTIMONY

The substance is dissolved in a solution of sodium potassium tartrate with gentle heating and cooled. Sodium sulphide solution is added drop by drop to this solution.A reddish-orange precipitate is produced and it dissolves on the addition of sodium hydroxide solution.

ARSENIC

An aqueous solution of the substance is heated on a water bath with an equal volume of hypophosphorus reagent. A brown precipitate is formed.

BARIUM

1. In the flame test, barium salts burn in a nonluminous flame with a yellowish -green colour. It appears blue when viewed through a green glass.
2. The substance is dissolved in dilute hydrochloric acid and dilute sulphuric acid is added. A white precipitate (of barium sulphate) is formed. It is insoluble in nitric acid.

BISMUTH

1. Dilute hydrochloric acid is added to the substance and boiled and cooled. It is diluted with water. A white or slightly yellow precipitate (of bismuth oxychloride) is formed. Sodium sulphide solution is added to this. The colour of the precipitate turns brown (due to the formation of bismuth sulphide).
2. Dilute nitric acid is added to an aqueous solution of the substance, heated to boiling and cooled. When thiourea solution is added to this, an orange yellow colour or an orange precipitate is produced. Sodium fluoride solution is now added. The solution is not decolourised within thirty minutes.

CALCIUM

1. Solutions of calcium salts in acetic acid give no precipitate when potassiuim ferrocyanide solution is added. However, on adding ammonium chloride, a white, crystalline precipitate is formed.

2. Solutions of calcium salts give, with ammonium oxalate solution, a white precipitate (of calcium oxalate) which is soluble in hydrochloric acid but sparingly soluble in acetic acid.

3. Calcium salts, dissolved in hydrochloric acid and neutralised with sodium hydroxide, give with ammonium carbonate solution a white precipitate (of calcium carbonate) which, after boiling and cooling, is insoluble in ammonium chloride solution.

IRON

I. Ferric Salts

1. To an aqueous solution of a ferric salt is added potassium ferrocyanide solution. An intense blue precipitate is produced. It is insoluble in dilute hydrochloric acid.

2. To an aqueous solution of a ferric salt, add dilute hydrochloric acid and ammonium thiocyanate solution. It becomes blood-red (ferric thiocyanate) in colour. Divide into two portions. Extract one with solvent ether. The ether layer is pink. To the other add mercuric chloride solution. The colour disappears.

3. Solution of a ferric salt, strongly acidified with acetic acid, gives with a 0.2 per cent solution of 7-iodo-8-hydroxyquinoline-5-sulphonic acid a stable green colour.

II. Ferrous Salts

1. To an aqueous solution of a ferrous salt, dilute sulphuric acid and solution of 1,10-phenanthroline are added. An intense red colour is produced. It is discharged when ceric ammonium sulphate solution is added.

2. Solution of a ferrous salt gives with potassium ferricyanide solution a dark blue precipitate. It is insoluble in dilute

hydrochloric acid. But it is decomposed by sodium hydroxide solution.

3. Solution of a ferrous salt gives with potassium ferrocyanide solution a white precipitate. This rapidly turns blue. It is also insoluble in dilute hydrochloric acid.

LEAD

1. Solution of a lead salt in acetic acid gives with potassium chromate solution a yellow precipitate of lead chromate. It is insoluble in sodium hydroxide solution.

2. Solution of a lead salt in acetic acid diluted with water, gives with potassium iodide solution a yellow precipitate. It is heated to boiling and allowed to cool. The precipitate is reformed as yellow, glistening plates (golden spangles of lead iodide).

MAGNESIUM

1. An aqueous solution of the substance gives a white precipitate (magnesium hydroxide) on adding ammonia. When ammonium chloride is added, it dissolves. When disodium hydrogen phosphate solution is added, a white crystalline precipitate (magnesium ammonium phosphate) is formed.

2. Titan yellow solution and sodium hydroxide solution are added to an aqueous solution of the substance. A bright red turbidity appears. It is gradually changed to a bright red precipitate.

MERCUROUS AND MERCURIC SALTS

I. Reactions Common to Mercurous and Mercuric Salts.

1. Hydrogen sulphide produces a black precipitate which is insoluble in ammonium sulphide solution and in boiling nitric acid.

2. Dissolve the mercurous or mercuric salt in nitric acid avoiding excess of acid. Immerse a bright copper foil in this solution. It gets coated with a deposit of mercury which on rubbing becomes bright. The foil may be heated and the mercury volatilised and obtained in the form of globules.

3. Stannous chloride added in excess to the solution of a mercurous or mercuric salt gives a white precipitate rapidly turning grey with excess of the reagent.

II. Reactions of Mercuric Salts

1. Solution of a mercuric salt gives with sodium hydroxide solution a yellow precipitate (yellow mercuric oxide is formed).

2. Solution of potassium iodide added to a neutral solution of a mercuric salt gives a scarlet precipitate (mercuric iodide). When more potassium iodide solution is added, the precipitate is soluble. It is also soluble in a large excess of the solution of the mercuric salt (finally a solution of potassium mercuri iodide is formed).

POTASSIUM

1. Solution of a potassium salt mixed with dilute acetic acid and a freshly prepared solution of sodium cobaltnitrite gives a yellow or orange-yellow precipitate immediately (a double salt of potassium sodium cobaltnitrite is formed).

2. No precipitate is formed when solution of a potassium salt is heated with sodium carbonate solution. Sodium sulphide solution is added. Still no precipitate is formed. It is cooled in ice water, tartaric acid solution is added and allowed to stand. A white crystalline precipitate is formed.

3. A small quantity of the substance is ignited and dissolved in water. To this platinic chloride solution and a little dilute hydrochloric acid are added. A yellow crystalline precipitate (of potassium chloroplatinate) is formed. When it is ignited, it leaves a residue of potassium chloride and platinum.

SILVER

1. Dilute hydrochloric acid is added to a solution of a silver salt. A curdy white precipitate (of silver chloride) is formed. It is insoluble in dilute ammonia. Potassium iodide solution is added. A yellow precipitate (of silver iodide) is formed.

2. Potassium chromate solution is added to a solution of a silver salt. A red precipitate (of silver chromate) is formed. It is soluble in nitric acid.

SODIUM

1. An aqueous solution of the substance is mixed with potassium carbonate solution and heated to boiling. No precipitate is formed. Freshly prepared potassium antimonate solution is now added and heated to boiling. It is allowed to cool in ice water and the inside of the test tube is rubbed with a glass rod. A dense, white precipitate is formed. It is disodium pyroantimonate, nearly insoluble in water, which is formed in a neutral or slightly alkaline solution.

2. The solution of the substance is acidified with dilute acetic acid and a large excess of magnesium uranylacetate solution is added, A yellow, crystalline precipitate (which is a triple acetate) is formed.

ZINC

1. An aqueous solution of a zinc salt is mixed with sodium hydroxide solution. A white precipitate (of zinc hydroxide) is formed. More sodium hydroxide solution is added. The precipitate redissolves (this is due to the formation of sodium zincate). Ammonium chloride solution is now added. The solution remains clear. Sodium sulphide solution is added. A flocculent, white precipitate is formed. This is due to the fact that ammonium sulphide (formed from ammonium chloride and sodium sulphide) precipitates white zinc sulphide from neutral, alkaline or faintly acid solution of a zinc salt.

2. Solutions of zinc salts, acidified with dilute sulphuric acid and mixed with one drop of very dilute copper sulphate solution and a small quantity of ammonium mercuri-thiocyanate solution, give a violet precipitate.

3. Solutions of zinc salts give with potassium ferrocyanide solution a white precipitate of zinc ferrocyanide. It is insoluble in dilute hyrochloric acid.

Section B
PRACTICAL

CHAPTER 14

IDENTIFICATION TESTS FOR SOME INORGANIC OFFICIAL COMPOUNDS

In Chapter 13 we studied about the official identification tests for cations and anions of the inorganic drugs and pharmaceuticals in a general way without going into practical details. In this Chapter we will take up some inorganic drugs and study the identification tests in detail including the tests for anions and cations in them. It is emphasised here that it is not necessary to do any systematic qualitative analysis followed by group analysis for identification of acidic and basic radicals in the inorganic substances as is the practice in pure chemistry. Our job is merely confined to finding out whether the substance is the same as that claimed on the label or not. For this purpose it is enough if we perform the identification tests given in the monograph of the drug in the pharmacopoeia and come to a conclusion.

The identification tests for some of the official inorganic drugs are discussed below. Along with the official tests some very useful non-official tests are also given:-

A. AMMONIUM CHLORIDE (I.P.1985)

Ammonium chloride gives the reactions of ammonium salts and of chlorides.

Reactions of Ammonium Salts

S.No.	Experiment	Observation	Inference
	Official Tests		
1.	Heat a few mg of the substance with sodium hydroxide solution.	Ammonia is evolved. It has a pungent, characteristic odour. It turns moist red litmus paper blue.	May be an ammonium salt.

186

S.No.	Experiment	Observation	Inference
2.	To a few ml of the solution of the substance add 0.2 g of light magnesium oxide. Pass the gas evolved into first beneath the surface of a mixture of 1ml of 0.1N hydrochloric acid and 0.05 ml of methyl red solution.	The colour of the solution changes to yellow from red.	
	Add 1 ml of a freshly prepared 10% w/v solution of sodium cobaltnitrite.	A yellow precipitate is formed.	May be an ammonium salt.
	Non-official Test		
3.	Add 1 ml of Nessler's reagent to 0.5 ml of the solution of the substance.	A yellow to brown colour is formed.	May be an ammonium salt.

Reactions of Chlorides

Official Tests

1.	Dissolve about 5 mg of the substance in 2 ml of water. Acidify with dilute nitric acid and add 0.5 ml of silver nitrate solution. Shake and allow to stand.	A curdy, white precipitate is formed.	
	Divide the precipitate into two portions. To one portion add conc. nitric acid.	The precipitate is not dissolved.	
	To the other portion add dilute ammonia solution.	The precipitate is dissolved.	

187

S.No.	Experiment	Observation	Inference
	Add a little conc.nitric acid to the second portion above.	The curdy, white precipitate is again formed.	May be a chloride.
	To about 10 mg of the substance, add 0.2 g of potassium dichromate and 1 ml of conc. sulphuric acid. Place a filter paper moistened with 0.1 ml of diphenyl-carbazide solution over the opening of the test tube.	The diphenyl-carbazide paper turns violet - red.	May be a chloride.

B. SODIUM BICARBONATE (I.P.1985)

Sodium bicarbonate answers the reactions of sodium and of bicarbonates.

Reactions of Sodium

S.No.	Experiment	Observation	Inference
	Official Tests		
1.	Dissolve 0.1g of the substance in 2 ml of water, add 2 ml of a 15% w/v solution of pot.carbonate and heat to boiling.	No precipitate is formed.	
	Add 4 ml of a freshly prepared solution of potassium antimonate and heat to boiling. Allow to cool in ice water and rub the inside of the test tube with a glass rod, if necessary.	A dense white precipitate is formed.	May be a sodium salt.

188

S.No.	Experiment	Observation	Inference
2.	Take a solution of the substance and acidify with N acetic acid. Add a large excess of magnesium uranyl-acetate solution.	A yellow, crystalline precipitate is formed.	May be a sodium salt.

Non-official Tests

S.No.	Experiment	Observation	Inference
3.	Repeat Test No.2 above with hydrochloric acid and cobalt uranyl-acetate.	A golden yellow precipitate is formed.	May be a sodium salt.
4.	**Flame Test:** Moisten a small quantity of the substance with enough concentrated hydrochloric acid to make a paste. Introduce a little of this paste on a platinum wire into the nonluminous flame of a Bunsen burner.	It burns with a golden yellow colour.	May be a sodium salt.

Reactions of Bicarbonates

Official Tests:

S.No.	Experiment	Observation	Inference
1.	Boil a solution of the substance and pass the gas evolved into clear lime water (distinction from carbonates).	Lime water turns milky..	May be a bicarbonate.
2.	Add magnesium sulphate solution to the solution of the substance (distinction from carbonates).	No precipitate is formed.	May be a bicarbonate.
	Boil the solution.	A white precipitate is formed.	May be a bicarbonate.

S.No.	Experiment	Observation	Inference
3.	Dissolve 0.1 g of the substance in sufficient water and add 2 ml of 2N acetic acid. Close the tube with a stopper fitted with a L-tube. Heat gently and pass the gas evolved into 5 ml of barium hydroxide solution.	A white precipitate is formed.	May be a bicarbonate.
	Add an excess of dilute hydrochloric acid.	The precipitate is dissolved.	May be a bicarbonate.
	Non-official Tests		
4.	To a little of the substance in a test tube, add dilute hydrochloric acid. Pass the gas evolved into lime water.	Lime water turns milky.	May be a bicarbonate or carbonate.
5.	Take 0.1 g of the substance and dissolve in water. Add 0.5 ml of mercuric chloride solution.	A white precipitate is formed.	May be a bicarbonate

C. SODIUM THIOSULPHATE (I.P.1985)

Sodium thiosulphate answers the reactions of sodium and thiosulphate. **For reactions of sodium, refer sodium bicarbonate.**

Reactions of Thiosulphates

S.No.	Experiment	Observation	Inference
1.	Dissolve 0.1 g of the substance in 5 ml of water and add 2 ml of concentrated hydro-chloric acid.	A white precipitate, soon turning yellow, is formed. Sulphur dioxide is evolved.	May be a thiosulphate.

S.No.	Experiment	Observation	Inference
2.	Dissolve 0.1 g of the substance in 5 ml of water and add 2 ml of Ferric Chloride T.S.	A dark violet colour is produced. It quickly disappears.	May be a thiosulphate.
3.	Take a small quantity of iodine solution in a test tube and add the sodium thiosulphate solution.	The colour of the iodine solution is discharged.	
	Add a little dilute hydrochloric acid and dilute sulphuric acid.	No white precipitate is formed.	May be a thiosulphate.
4.	Add the sodium thiosulphate solution to bromine solution.	Bromine is decolourised.	
	Add a little dilute hydrochloric acid and dilute sulphuric acid.	A white precipitate is formed.	May be a thiosulphate.

D. SODIUM NITRITE (I.P.1966)

Sodium nitrite answers the reactions of sodium and of nitrites.

For reactions of sodium, refer under sodium bicarbonate.

Reactions of Nitrites

S.No.	Experiment	Observation	Inference
1.	Heat 0.1 g of the substance with dilute sulphuric acid.	Red fumes are evolved.	May be a nitrite.
2.	Dissolve 0.1 g of the substance in water and add a few drops of dilute sulphuric acid, potassium iodide solution and starch solution.	A blue colour is produced.	May be a nitrite.

191

S.No.	Experiment	Observation	Inference
3.	Dissolve 0.1 g of the substance in water and add 1 ml of ferrous sulphate solution.	A deep brown colour is produced.	May be a nitrite.
4.	Dissolve 0.1 g of the substance in water and add 0.1 g of urea and 1 ml of dilute sulphuric acid. Pass the evolved carbon dioxide gas into calcium hydroxide solution.	Calcium hydroxide solution (lime water) turns milky.	May be a nitrite.

E. DICALCIUM PHOSPHATE (I.P.1985)

Dicalcium phosphate or dibasic calcium phosphate answers the reactions of calcium and of phosphates with some pretreatment.

Reactions of Calcium

S.No.	Experiment	Observation	Inference
	Official Tests		
	Pretreatment: Take 0.1 g of the substance, add 5 ml of water and 5 ml of dilute hydrochloric acid and warm till it dissolves. Use this solution for the reactions given below:		
1.	Take 5 ml of the solution and add 1 ml of glacial acetic acid.	The solution remains clear.	
	Add 0.5 ml of potassium ferrocyanide solution. Add about 50 mg of ammonium chloride	A white, crystalline precipitate is formed.	May be a calcium salt.

S.No.	Experiment	Observation	Inference
2.	To 1 ml of solution, add a few drops of ammonium oxalate.	A white precipitate is produced.	
	Divide into two portions. To one portion add a little dilute acetic acid.	The precipitate is not dissolved.	
	To the other portion add concentrated hydrochloric acid.	The precipitate is dissolved.	May be a calcium salt.
3.	Take 5 ml of the solution and neutralise the solution with dilute sodium hydroxide solution. Add 5 ml of ammonium carbonate solution.	A white precipitate is formed.	
	Boil and cool the mixture. Add 2 ml of ammonium chloride solution.	The precipitate is not dissolved.	May be a calcium salt.
	Non-official Tests		
4.	Mix a little of the substance with enough concentrated hydrochloric acid to make a paste. Introduce a little of this on a platinum wire into a Bunsen flame.	A brick red colour is seen.	May be a calcium salt.
5.	To a concentrated solution of the substance add dilute sulphuric acid.	A white precipitate is produced.	May be a calcium salt.

S.No.	Experiment	Observation	Inference
6.	To a concentrated solution of the substance add potassium chromate solution.	A yellow crystalline precipitate is formed.	
	Divide into two portions. To one portion add water.	The precipitate dissolves.	
	To the other portion add dilute acetic acid.	The precipitate dissolves.	May be a calcium salt.

Reactions of Phosphates

Official Tests

Pretreatment:
Dissolve 0.1 g of the substance in a slight excess of warm dilute nitric acid. Reserve this solution for the reactions given below:

1.	Neutralise 5 ml of the above solution using dilute sodium hydroxide solution and a neutral point indicator like phenol red. To this add 5 ml of silver nitrate solution.	A light yellow precipitate is formed.	
	Divide into two portions. To one portion add dilute ammonia solution. To the other portion add dilute nitric acid.	The precipitate is dissolved.	May be a phosphate.

S.No.	Experiment	Observation	Inference
2.	To 1 ml of the solution add 1 ml of ammoniacal magnesium sulphate solution.	A white crystalline precipitate is produced.	May be a phosphate.
3.	Take 2 ml of the solution, add 2 ml of dilute nitric acid and 4 ml of ammonium molybdate solution and warm.	A bright, canary yellow precipitate is produced.	May be a phosphate.

F. MAGNESIUM CARBONATE (I.P.1985)

Magnesium carbonate occurs as either heavy magnesium carbonate or light magnesium carbonate. Either one of them can be used. Magnesium carbonate answers the reactions of magnesium and of carbonates.

Reactions of Magnesium

S.No.	Experiment	Observation	Inference
	Official Tests		
	Pretreatment: Dissolve about 0.2 g of the substance in dilute nitric acid. Copious effervescence is produced. Reserve this solution for the following tests:		
1.	To 2 ml of the above solution add 1 ml of dilute ammonia solution. Dissolve the white precipitate formed by adding 1 ml of 2M ammonium chloride. Finally add 1 ml of 0.25 M disodium hydrogen phosphate.	A white, crystalline precipitate is formed.	May be a magnesium salt.

S.No.	Experiment	Observation	Inference
2.	Neutralise 5 ml of the solution using phenol red as indicator. To this solution add 0.2 ml of a 0.1 per cent w/v solution of titan yellow and 0.5 ml of 0.1N sodium hydroxide.	A bright red turbidity develops. It is finally changed to a bright red precipitate.	May be a magnesium salt.

Non-official Tests

S.No.	Experiment	Observation	Inference
3.	Neutralise 1 ml of the solution and add 1 ml of ammonium carbonate solution.	A white precipitate is produced.	
	Add 1 ml of ammonium chloride solution.	The precipitate is dissolved.	May be a magnesium salt.
4.	To 1 ml of the solution add excess of sodium hydroxide solution.	A white precipitate is formed.	
	Add 2 ml of ammonium chloride solution.	The precipitate is dissolved.	May be a magnesium salt.
5.	To 1 ml of the solution add 1 ml of sodium hydroxide solution and 1 ml of diphenylcar-bazide solution.	A pink precipitate is produced.	May be a magnesium salt.

Reactions of Carbonates

Official Tests

S.No.	Experiment	Observation	Inference
1.	To 0.1 g of the substance in 2 ml of water add 2 ml of 2N acetic acid. Close the tube with a L-tube. Heat gently and collect the gas in 5 ml of 0.1 N barium hydroxide.	A white precipitate is formed.	

S.No.	Experiment	Observation	Inference
	Add an excess of dilute hydrochloric acid.	The precipitate is dissolved.	May be a carbonate.
2.	To the solution of the substance add a solution of magnesium sulphate.	A white precipitate is formed.	May be a carbonate.
	Non-official Tests		
3.	To 0.5 ml of the solution add 1 ml of mercuric chloride solution.	A brownish red precipitate is produced.	May be a carbonate.
4.	To 0.1 g of the substance in water add dilute hydrochloric acid. Pass the CO_2 gas produced into lime water.	Lime water turns milky.	May be a carbonate.

G. MAGNESIUM SULPHATE (I.P.1985)

A 1 in 20 (1 g in 20 ml) solution of magnesium sulphate gives the reactions of magnesium and of sulphates.

Reactions of Magnesium: Refer under magnesium carbonate.

Reactions of Sulphates:		
Official Tests		
1. To 5 ml of the solution, add 1ml of dilute hydrochloric acid and 1 ml of barium chloride solution.	A white precipitate is formed.	May be a sulphate.
2. To 5 ml of the solution add 2 ml of lead acetate solution.	A white precipitate is formed.	
Divide into two portions. To one portion add an excess of ammonium acetate solution.	The precipitate dissolves.	

197

S.No.	Experiment	Observation	Inference
	To the other portion add an excess of sodium hydroxide solution.	The precipitate dissolves.	May be sulphate.
3.	To the suspension obtained in test (1) add 0.1 ml of iodine solution.	The suspension is coloured yellow (distinction from sulphites and dithionites).	
	Add drop by drop stannous chloride solution.	The yellow colour is discharged (distinction from iodates).	
	Boil the mixture.	No coloured precipitate is formed (distinction from selenates and tungstates).	May be a sulphate.

H. ZINC OXIDE (I.P.1985)

A solution of zinc oxide in dilute hydrochloric acid gives the reactions of zinc in addition to answering test no (1) mentioned below.

S.No.	Experiment	Observation	Inference
1.	Heat about 1 g of the substance strongly.	It becomes yellow.	
	Cool the heated substance.	The yellow colour disappears.	May be zinc oxide.
	Pretreatment		
	Take about 1 g of the substance and add 20 ml of dilute hydrochloric acid. A solution is formed.		

S.No.	Experiment	Observation	Inference
2.	To 5 ml of the above solution add 0.2 ml of sodium hydroxide solution.	A white precipitate is formed.	
	Add another 2 ml of sodium hydroxide solution.	The precipitate is dissolved.	
	Add 10 ml of ammonium chloride solution.	There is no precipitation.	
	Add 0.1 ml of sodium sulphide solution.	A flocculent, white precipitate is formed.	May be a zinc salt.
3.	Acidify 5 ml of the solution with dilute sulphuric acid. Add one drop of a 0.1% w/v copper sulphate solution and 2 ml of ammonium mercurithiocyanate solution.	A violet precipitate is formed.	May be a zinc salt.
4.	To 5 ml of the solution add 2 ml of potassium ferrocyanide solution.	A white precipitate is formed.	
	Add 3 ml of dilute hydrochloric acid.	The precipitate is not dissolved.	May be a zinc salt.

I. ZINC SULPHATE (I.P.1985)

A 1 in 20 solution of zinc sulphate in water gives the reactions of zinc and of sulphates.

Reactions of Zinc: Refer under zinc oxide.

Reactions of Sulphates: Refer under magnesium sulphate

J. FERROUS SULPHATE (I.P.1985)

Ferrous sulphate gives the reactions of ferrous salts and of sulphates. A 1 in 20 solution of ferrous sulphate in water is used for this purpose.

Reactions of Ferrous Salts

Official Tests

S.No.	Experiment	Observation	Inference
	Pretreatment: Dissolve 0.5 g of the substance in 10 ml of water and reserve it for the following tests:-		
1.	Take 2 ml of the solution and add 2 ml of dilute sulphuric acid and 1 ml of a 0.1% w/v 1:10–phenanthroline solution.	An intense red colour is produced.	
	Ad a slight excess of 0.1N ceric ammonium sulphate.	The colour disappears.	May be a ferrous salt.
2.	Take 1 ml of the solution and add 1 ml of potassium ferricyanide solution.	A dark blue precipitate is formed.	
	Divide into two portions. To one portion add dilute hydrochloric acid.	The precipitate is not dissolved.	
	To the other portion add sodium hydroxide solution.	The precipitate is decomposed.	May be a ferrous salt.

S.No.	Experiment	Observation	Inference
3.	Take 1 ml of the solution and add 1 ml of potassium ferrocyanide solution.	A white precipitate is produced. It rapidly becomes blue.	
	Add dilute hydrochloric acid.	The precipitate is insoluble.	May be a ferrous salt.

Reactions of Sulphates: Refer under magnesium sulphate.

K. ALUM (I.P.1966)

Alum gives the reactions characteristic of aluminium, potassium and sulphates.

Reactions of Aluminium

S.No.	Experiment	Observation	Inference
	Official Tests		
1.	To 20 mg of the substance add 0.5 ml of 2N hydrochloric acid and 0.5 ml of thioacetamide reagent. Add 2N sodium hydroxide drop by drop.	A gelatinous, white precipitate is produced.	
	Add an excess of sodium hydroxide solution.	The precipitate is dissolved.	
	Gradually add 2N ammonium chloride solution.	The gelatinous white precipitate is again formed.	May be an aluminium salt.
2.	Dissolve 20 mg of the substance in water. Add dilute ammonia solution till a faint precipitate is produced.		

S.No.	Experiment	Observation	Inference
	Then add 0.25 ml of a freshly prepared solution of quinalizarin in 1% sodium hydroxide. Heat to boiling, cool and acidify with an excess of dilute acetic acid.	A reddish violet colour is produced	May be an aluminium salt.

Reactions of Potassium

Official Tests

S.No.	Experiment	Observation	Inference
1.	Dissolve 50 mg in 1 ml of water and add 1 ml of dilute acetic acid and 1 ml of a freshly prepared 10% solution of sodium cobaltnitrite.	A yellow or orange-yellow precipitate is formed immediately.	May be a potassium salt.
2.	Dissolve 0.1 g of the substance in 2 ml of water and add 1 ml of sodium carbonate solution and heat.	No precipitate is formed.	
	Add 0.5 ml of sodium sulphide solution.	No precipitate is formed.	
	Cool in ice water, add 2 ml of 15% tartaric acid solution and allow to stand.	A white crystalline precipitate is formed.	May be a potassium salt.
3.	Ignite a small quantity of the substance and dissolve in minimum quantity of water. To this solution add 1 ml of platinic chloride solution and 1 ml of concentrated hydrochloric acid.	A yellow crystalline precipitate is formed.	May be a potassium salt.

Reactions of Sulphates: Refer under magnesium sulphate.

L. POTASSIUM IODIDE (I.P.1985)

A 1 in 20 solution of potassium iodide in water gives the reactions of potassium and of iodides.

Reactions of Potassium: Refer under Alum.

Reactions of Iodides

Official Tests

Pretreatment: Dissolve 0.5 g of the substance in 10 ml of water and reserve it for the following tests.

S.No.	Experiment	Observation	Inference
1.	Take 2 ml of the solution and acidify it with dilute nitric acid. Add 0.5 ml of silver nitrate solution. Shake and allow to stand.	A curdy, pale yellow precipitate is formed.	
	Add 2 ml of dilute ammonia.	The precipitate is not dissolved.	May be an iodide.
2.	To 0.2 ml of the solution add 0.5 ml of dilute sulphuric acid, 0.2 ml of potassium dichromate solution, 2 ml of water and 2 ml of chloroform. Shake for half a minute and allow to stand.	The chloroform layer is coloured violet or violet-red.	May be an iodide.
3.	To 1 ml of the solution add 0.5 ml of mercuric chloride.	A dark red precipitate is formed.	
	Add an excess of potassium iodide solution.	The precipitate dissolves and a clear solution is formed.	May be an iodide.

S.No.	Experiment	Observation	Inference
	Non-official Tests		
4.	To 1 ml of the solution add 1 ml of dilute acetic acid, 1 ml of potassium iodate solution and 0.5 ml of starch solution.	A blue colour is formed.	May be an iodide.
5.	To 1 ml of the solution add 1 ml of chlorine solution and 1 ml of chloroform.	The chloroform layer is coloured violet or violet-red.	May be an iodide.

List of Some Other Substances for which Identification Tests can be done

I.P.1985

1. Calcium Carbonate
2. Calcium Gluconate
3. Sodium Chloride
4. Sodium Citrate
5. Sodium Salicylate

I.P.1966

1. Ammoniated Mercury
2. Borax
3. Yellow Mercuric Oxide.

CHAPTER 15
LIMIT TESTS

Limit tests are quantitative or semi-quantitative tests which are designed to detect and control small quantities of impurities which are likely to be present in the substance.

These tests require a standard containing a definite amount of impurity to be set up at the same time and under the same conditions of the test experiment. In this way, it is possible to compare the amount of the impurity in the substance with a standard of known concentration and find out whether the impurity is within or excess of the limit prescribed.

For this purpose these tests make use of simple comparisons of opalescence, turbidity or colour with standards as prescribed in the pharmacopoeias. By taking different quantities of the test substance it is possible to vary the limits of the impurities permitted for each substance. No numerical values are given for the permitted limits because other impurities also may interfere with the tests. Variations in time and method of performing the tests also influence the tests.

Limit Test for Chlorides (I.P.1985)

Aim: To perform the limit test for chlorides on the given sample labelled as Dextrose I.P. and report on its standard.

Principle: The limit test for chlorides is based on the well-known reaction between silver nitrate and soluble chlorides forming a precipitate of silver chloride which is insoluble in dilute nitric acid. The opalescence produced depends upon the amount of chlorides present in the sample. It is compared with the opalescence produced in a standard solution containing the prescribed quantity of chloride similarly treated. If the opalescence in the sample is less than that in the standard, it passes the test and is declared as standard. The test is done in Nessler cylinders.

$$Cl^- + AgNO_3 \rightarrow AgCl\downarrow + NO_{3-}$$

Procedure: Take two 50 ml Nessler cylinders. Label one as "Test" and the other as "Standard".

Test	Standard
1. Dissolve the specified quantity of the substance (1 g of dextrose) in distilled water or prepare a solution as directed in the text in the Nessler cylinder.	Pipette out 1 ml of a 0.05845 per cent w/v solution of sodium chloride into the Nessler cylinder.
2. Add 10 ml of dilute nitric acid.	Add 10 ml of dilute nitric acid.
3. Dilute to 50 ml with water.	Dilute to 50 ml with water.
4. Add 1 ml of silver nitrate solution.	Add 1 ml of silver nitrate solution.
5. Stir immediately with a glass rod and allow to stand for five minutes.	Stir immediately with a glass rod and allow to stand for 5 minutes.

Observation: Observe whether the test has a greater opalescence than the standard or lesser opalescence than the standard. Write *one* of the following:

1. When viewed transversely, the opalescence produced in the test is not greater than the standard opalescence.

2. When viewed transversely, the opalescence produced in the test is greater than the standard opalescence.

Report: Write *either one* for the following according to the observation that you got:

1. The sample (of dextrose) passes the test. As far as this limit test is concerned, it is standard.

2. The sample (of dextrose) does not pass the test. As far as this limit test is concerned, it is substandard.

List of Some Substances for which Limit Test for Chlorides is Prescribed in I.P.1985

1. Calcium carbonate

2. Calcium gluconate
3. Calcium hydroxide
4. Calcium lactate
5. Dextrose.
6. Heavy magnesium carbonate
7. Light magnesium carbonate
8. Heavy magnesium oxide
9. Light magnesium oxide
10. Magnesium sulphate
11. Potassium citrate
12. Sodium acetate
13. Sodium acid phosphate
14. Sodium benzoate
15. Sodium bicarbonate
16. Sodium citrate
17. Sodium phosphate
18. Sodium salicylate
19. Sodium thiosulphate
20. Urea
21. Zinc sulphate.

Limit Test for Sulphates (I.P.1985)

Aim: To perform the limit test for sulphates on the given sample labelled as Sodium Chloride, I.P. and report on its standard.

Principle: The limit test for sulphates is based on the reaction between barium chloride and soluble sulphates in the presence of dilute hydrochloric acid. The turbidity produced in the test is compared with the turbidity produced in a standard containing a known quantity of sulphate and similarly treated. Barium sulphate reagent which contains barium chloride, sulphate-free alcohol and a small quantity of potassium sulphate is used as the reagent. The inclusion of the small quantity of potassium sulphate in the reagent increases the sensitivity of the test. Alcohol prevents supersaturation and a more uniform turbidity develops. The test substance passes the test if the turbidity produced in it is not greater than the turbidity produced in the standard. If the turbidity in the test is greater, it fails the test.

$$SO_4^{--} + BaCl_2 \rightarrow BaSO_4\downarrow + 2Cl^-$$

Procedure: Take two 50 ml Nessler cylinders. Label one as "Test" and the other as "Standard".

Test	Standard
1. Dissolve the specified quantity of the substance (2 g of sodium chloride) in water or prepare a solution as directed in the text in the Nessler cylinder.	Pipette out 1 ml of a 0.1089 per cent w/v solution of potassium sulphate into the Nessler cylinder.
2. Add 2 ml of dilute hydrochloric acid.	Add 2 ml of dilute hydrochloric acid.
3. Dilute to 45 ml with water.	Dilute to 45 ml with water.
4. Add 5 ml of barium sulphate reagent.	Add 5 ml of barium sulphate reagent.
5. Stir immediately with a glass rod and allow to stand for 5 minutes.	Stir immediately with a glass rod and allow to stand for 5 minutes.

Observations: Observe whether the turbidity produced in the test is greater than the standard turbidity and write *either one* of the following:

1. When viewed transversely, the turbidity produced in the test is not greater than the standard turbidity.

or

2. When viewed transversely, the turbidity produced in the test is greater than the standard turbidity.

Report: Write *either one* of the following according as you have the observation of (1) or (2).

1. The sample of the substance (sodium chloride) passes the test. It is standard for this test.

2. The sample of the substance (sodium chloride) does not pass the test. So it is substandard.

List of Some Substances for which Limit Test for Sulphates is Prescribed in I.P.1985

1. Calcium carbonate.
2. Calcium gluconate
3. Calcium hydroxide.
4. Anhydrous citric acid and citric acid
5. Dextrose
6. Heavy magnesium carbonate
7. Light magnesium carbonate
8. Heavy magnesium oxide
9. Light magnesium oxide
10. Potassium bromide
11. Potassium chloride
12. Potassium citrate.
13. Sodium acetate.
14. Sodium acid phosphate
15. Sodium benzoate
16. Sodium bicarbonate
17. Sodium chloride
18. Sodium citrate
19. Sodium phosphate
20. Sodium salicylate
21. Sodium thiosulphate
22. Urea.

Limit Test for Iron (I.P.1985)

Aim: To perform the limit test for iron on the given sample labelled as Sodium Chloride, I.P. and report on its standard.

Principle: The test depends upon the reaction between ferrous iron and thioglycollic acid in the presence of ammonia when a pale pink to deep reddish purple colour is produced. Ferric iron is reduced to ferrous iron by the thioglycollic acid and the compound produced is ferrous thioglycollate. Citric acid forms a soluble complex with iron and pre vents its precipitation by ammonia as ferrous hydroxide. Ferrous thio glycollate is colourless in neutral or acid solutions. The colour develops only in the presence of alkali. It is stable in the absence of air but fades when exposed to air due to oxidation to the ferric compound. Therefore the colours should be compared immediately after the time allowed for full development of colour is over. The following reactions take place:

$$2Fe^{+++} + 2CH_2SH.COOH \rightarrow 2Fe^{++} + S.CH_2.COOH$$

Ferric	Thioglycollic	Ferrous	
iron	acid	Iron	S.CH_2 COOH

$+2H^+$

$$Fe^{++} + 2CH_2SH.COOH \rightarrow$$

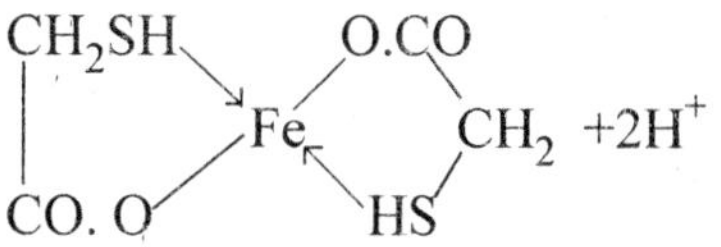

$$\begin{array}{c} CH_2SH \qquad O.CO \\ | \qquad \qquad \diagdown Fe \diagup \qquad CH_2 \quad +2H^+ \\ CO.O \diagup \qquad \diagdown HS \end{array}$$

Ferrous thioglycollate

Procedure: Take two 50 ml Nessler cylinders. Label one as "Test" and the other as "Standard".

	Test	Standard
1.	Dissolve a specified quantity of the substance (1 g of sodium chloride) in 40 ml of water or use 10 ml of the solution as prescribed in the monograph and transfer to a Nessler cylinder.	Dilute 2 ml of standard iron solution with 40 ml of water in a Nessler cylinder.
2.	Add 2 ml of a 20% w/v solution of iron-free citric acid and 0.1 ml of thioglycollic acid and mix.	Add 2 ml of a 20% w/v solution of iron-free citric acid and 0.1 ml of thioglycollic acid and mix.
3.	Make alkaline with iron-free ammonia solution.	Make alkaline with iron-free ammonia solution.
4.	Dilute to 50 ml with water.	Dilute to 50 ml with water.
5.	Allow to stand for 5 minutes.	Allow to stand for five minutes.

Observation: Observe whether the colour produced in the test is not more intense than the standard colour and write *either one* of the following:

1. The colour produced in the test is not more intense than the standard colour.

2. The colour produced in the test is more intense than the standard colour.

Report: Write *either one* of the following according as you have the observation of (1) or (2);

1. The sample (of sodium chloride) passes the test. so it is standard for this test.

2. The sample (of sodium chloride) does not pass the test. So it is substandard.

List of Some Substances for which Limit Test for Iron is Prescribed in I.P.1985

1. Calcium carbonate
2. Calcium chloride
3. Calcium lactate
4. Dibasic calcium phosphate
5. Tribasic calcium phosphate
6. Glycerin
7. Lactic acid
8. Heavy magnesium carbonate
9. Light magnesium carbonate
10. Heavy magnesium oxide
11. Light magnesium oxide
12. Magnesium sulphate
13. Magnesium trisilicate
14. Phosphoric acid
15. Potassium bromide
16. Potassium chloride
17. Procaine hydrochloride
18. Sodium acetate
19. Sodium bicarbonate
20. Sodium chloride

21. Zinc oxide
22. Zinc sulphate

Limit Test for Heavy Metals (I.P.1985)

This limit test is for detecting and limiting the impurity of heavy metals likely to be present in many drugs. The heavy metals are precipitated as their sulphides by the addition of either hydrogen sulphide or sodium sulphide solution under specified conditions. A dark brown to light brown colour is produced depending upon the amount of heavy metals present. This is compared with the colour produced in a standard prepared by taking a specified quantity of standard lead solution and similarly treating it. The test solution and the standard solution are prepared in 50 ml Nessler cylinders and are diluted to the mark. Since many heavy metals are likely to be present, lead is chosen as the standard to represent all the heavy metals.

The precipitation is carried out at a pH of 3 to 4 by adjustment with dilute acetic acid for substances which are precipitated as their sulphides in moderately acid conditions (Method A). Organic compounds like benzocaine or lactic acid or paracetamol should be treated specially with mineral acids and ignited to destroy organic matter. The residue is extracted with hot water and adjusted to a pH of 3 to 4 as in Method A and the limit test is done on this solution containing the extracted heavy metals as in Method A(Method B). When no clear solution can be obtained with the test substance (eg. acetazolamide) by dissolving in acid as under Method A or Method B, the substance may be dissolved in sodium hydroxide solution for obtaining a clear solution. Using this solution the limit test is done under alkaline conditions. Almost all the heavy metals are precipitated under these conditions as their sulphides (Method C).

If 2 ml of standard lead solution is taken for preparing the standard solution and 1 g of the test substance is taken for preparing the test solution, then the heavy meals limit prescribed is 20 parts per million. Standard lead solution contains 0.01 mg of lead per ml and should be freshly prepared. If 0.5 g of the test substance is used, then the limit prescribed is 40 parts per million. Similarly if 2 g of the test substance are taken, the limit permitted is 10 parts per million. All reagents used should be free from heavy metals and are designated as Sp.

Aim: To perform the limit test for heavy metals on the given sample labelled as Boric Acid, I.P. and report on its standard.

Principle: This limit test is for detecting and limiting the impurity of heavy metals. The heavy metals are precipitated as their sulphides by the addition of hydrogen sulphide or sodium sulphide solution. The sample is dissolved in acid or alkali for making a solution. If acid is used, the pH is adjusted to a value of 3 to 4 by adding either dilute acetic acid or dilute ammonia solution. The test is done in two 50 ml Nessler cylinders. The test solution is prepared in one cylinder and a standard solution is prepared in the other cylinder taking the prescribed volume of standard lead solution. The reagent solution is then added to both and they are diluted to the mark and mixed. After standing for five minutes, they are compared.

Procedure: Take two 50 ml Nessler cylinders. Label one as 'Test Solution' and the other as 'Standard Solution'.

	Test Solution	Standard Solution
1.	Place 25 ml of the solution prepared for the test as directed in the individual monograph (for boric acid, dissolve 1 g of sample in 2 ml of dilute acetic acid and add enough distilled water to make up to 25 ml) in the Nessler cylinder.	Pipette out 2 ml of standard lead solution into the Nessler cylinder and dilute with distilled water to 25 ml.
2.	Adjust with either dilute acetic acid Sp or dilute ammonia solution Sp to a pH between 3 and 4.	Adjust with either dilute acetic acid Sp or dilute ammonia solution Sp to a pH between 3 and 4.
3.	Dilute with water to about 35 ml and mix.	Dilute with water to about 35 ml and mix.
4.	Add 10 ml of freshly prepared hydrogen sulphide solution and mix.	Add 10 ml of freshly prepared hydrogen sulphide solution and mix.
5.	Dilute with water to 50 ml and allow to stand for five minutes.	Dilute with water to 50 ml and allow to stand for five minutes.

Observation: Observe whether the test solution has a darker colour than that of the standard and write *one* of the following:

1. When viewed downwards over a white surface, the colour produced in the test solution is not darker than that produced in the standard solution.

2. When viewed downwards over a white surface, the colour produced in the test solution is darker than that produced in the standard solution.

Report: Write *one* of the following reports according to the observation made:

1. The sample passes the limit test. So it is standard for this test.

2. The sample does not pass the limit test. So it is substandard.

List of Some Substances for which Limit Test for Heavy Metals is Prescribed in I.P.1985

Method A

Aluminium hydroxide gel
Dried aluminium hydroxide gel
Aluminium sulphate
Aminophylline
Ammonium chloride
Analgin
Ascorbic acid
Barium sulphate
Boric acid
Calcium chloride
Calcium gluconate
Calcium hydroxide
Calcium lactate
Calcium levulinate
Dibasic calcium phosphate
Tribasic calcium phosphate
Citric acid
Anhydrous citric acid

Dextrose
Glycerin
Lactose
Milk of magnesia
Magnesium chloride
Magnesium sulphate
Phosphoric acid
Potassium bromide
Potassium chloride
Potassium citrate
Potassium iodide
Sodium acetate
Sodium acid phosphate
Sodium benzoate
Sodium bicarbonate
Sodium chloride
Sodium hydroxide
Sodium phosphate

Method B

Benzocaine
Calcium aminosalicylate
Microcrystalline cellulose
Chloroquine phosphate
Frusemide
Isoniazid
Lactic acid
Paracetamol
Saccharin
Sodium aminosalicylate
Sodium ascorbate

Method C

Acetazolamide
Quinalbarlbitone sodium

Limit Test for Arsenic (I.P.1985)

Aim: To perform the limit test for arsenic on the given sample labelled as Dextrose, I.P. and report on its standard.

Principle: The test substance is dissolved in hydrochloric acid or an aqueous solution or extract is acidified. Some substances have to be specially treated for making a solution suitable for the test. The arsenic present in the sample is converted to either arsenious acid or arsenic acid depending on its valency state. Then it is further treated with a reducing agent such as stannous chloride. Arsenic acid is reduced to arsenious acid. In the I.P., stannated hydrochloric acid (stannous chloride mixed with hydrochloric acid) is added to the substance.

$$H_3AsO_4 \rightarrow H_3AsO_3$$
Arsenic acid   Arsenious acid

Potassium iodide which is also added forms hydriodic acid which also reduces arsenic acid to arsenious acid.

The arsenious acid is further reduced to arsine by nascent hydrogen produced by the action of granulated zinc and hydrochloric acid.

$$H_3AsO_4 + 6H \rightarrow AsH_3\uparrow + 3H_2$$
Arsine

When arsine comes into contact with dry paper saturated with mercuric chloride, it produces a yellow stain.

$$2AsH_3 + HgCl_2 \rightarrow Hg{\overset{\displaystyle AsH_2}{\underset{\displaystyle AsH_2}{\big\langle}}} + 2HCl$$
Yellow or brown stain

The intensity of the stain is compared by daylight with a standard stain which is similarly and simultaneously prepared by taking a specified quantity of dilute arsenic solution in place of the test substance. If the test stain is less in intensity of colour than the standard stain, the sample passes the test.

All the reagents used excepting strong and dilute arsenic solutions should be arsenic-free and are designated as AsT. A standard stain prepared by taking 1 ml of dilute arsenic solution AsT and compared with the test stain produced by taking 10 g of the test substance indicates that the permitted limit of arsenic is 1 part per million.

Apparatus: The apparatus consists of a wide-mouthed glass bottle (about 120 ml capacity) fitted with a rubber bung. A glass tube of specified dimensions is passed through the rubber bung. The internal diameter of the tube (6.5 mm) is important and should be uniform throughout. The tube is open at the upper end but tapers to a small diameter at the lower end. Near the lower end a small hole is present to allow condensed moisture to escape.

The tube is packed lightly with cotton wool saturated with lead acetate solution and dried. This is to trap any hydrogen sulphide which may be produced during the reaction, if any sulphur impurity is present in the substance.

The mercuric chloride paper is fixed at the upper end of the tube between two rubber bungs by means of a spring clip. The two rubber

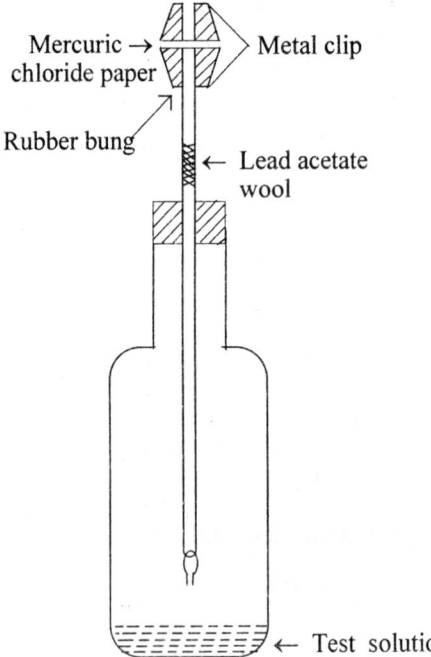

Apparatus for Limit Test for Arsenic

bungs contain the tube in two parts and the mercuric chloride paper is correctly positioned between them.

Procedure: Take two 120 ml wide-mouthed bottles with the attachments and label one as "Test" and the other as "standard".

	Test	Standard
1.	Weigh accurately 10 g of the sample and dissolve in 50 ml of water. Transfer to the bottle.	Take in the bottle accurately 1 ml of dilute arsenic solution. Add 50 ml of water.
2.	Add 10 ml of stannated hydrochloric acid AsT.	Add 10 ml of stannated hydrochloric acid AsT.
3.	Add 1 g of potassium iodide AsT and 10 g of zinc AsT.	Add 1 g of potassium iodide AsT and 10 g of zinc AsT.
4.	Place the cork immediately over the bottle with the attachments.	Place the cork with the attachments over the bottle.
5.	Allow the reaction to go on in the cold for forty minutes.	Allow the reaction to go on in the cold for forty minutes.
6.	Remove the mercuric chloride paper at the end of forty minutes.	Remove the mercuric chloride paper at the end of forty minutes.

Observation: Compare by daylight the depth of colour in the test stain with the standard stain. Report *either one* of the following:

1. The test stain has more depth of colour than the standard stain.,

or

2. The test stain has less depth of colour than the standard stain.

Report: Report *either one* of the following according to the observation:

1. The sample does not pass the test. It is substandard.

2. The sample passes the test. It is standard for the test.

List of Some Substances for Which Limit Test for Arsenic is Prescribed in I.P.1985

1. Aluminium
2. Ammonium chloride
3. Barium sulphate
4. Calcium chloride
5. Calcium gluconate
6. Calcium levulinate
7. Citric acid
8. Anhydous citric acid.
9. Dextrose
10. Glycerin
11. Hydrochloric acid
12. Heavy kaolin
13. Light kaolin
14. Lactic acid
15. Lactose
16. Magnesium chloride
17. Magnesium sulphate
18. Magnesium trisilicate
19. Potassium bromide
20. Potassium chloride
21. Potassium citrate
22. Potassium iodide
23. Sodium acetate
24. Sodium acid phosphate
25. Sodium chloride
26. Sodium citrate
27. Sodium phosphate
28. Sodium thiosulphate
29. Tartaric acid
30. Zinc sulphate.

CHAPTER 16

QUANTITATIVE ANALYSIS OF INORGANIC COMPOUNDS

Quantitative analysis means the estimation of the amount of a particular substance present in a sample. For this purpose several methods such as volumetric analysis, gravimetric analysis, instrumental methods of analysis etc. are used.

Volumetric Analysis

Volumetric analysis is also known as titrimetric analysis since this method involves the performance of titrations. In this analysis volumes of solutions of substances are reacted with volumes of solutions of other substances. For this purpose standard solutions of substances are used. A standard solution is one whose strength is accurately known. It contains a definite quantity of the substance in a definite volume of the solution.

Volumetric solutions can be prepared in different strengths or normalities. A **normal solution** is one which contains the equivalent weight of the substance in grams (one gram-equivalent weight) in one litre (1000 ml) of the solution. It is also known as 1N or $\frac{N}{1}$ solution. A **decinormal solution** is one which contains one-tenth of the gram equivalent weight ($\frac{1}{10}$) of the substance in one litre of the solution. It is also known as 0.1N or $\frac{N}{10}$ solution. Similarly a centinormal solution is one which contains one-hundredth ($\frac{N}{100}$) of the gram-equivalent weight of the substance in one litre of the solution.

A molar solution is one which contains one gram molecular weight of the substance in one litre of the solution. Molar solutions are used when equivalent weights for some substances are variable in different types of reactions.

Primary and Secondary Standards

The normality of a volumetric solution may be found out by two methods. In one method the substance can be accurately weighed and dissolved in water to make a definite volume of the solution. For example 63 grams of oxalic acid (accurately weighed) may be dissolved in water and made up to exactly 1000 ml to give a 1 N or $\frac{N}{1}$ solution. 63 grams is the gram equivalent weight of oxalic acid. Likewise 4.903 grams of potassium dichromate may be dissolved in water and made up to 1000 ml to give a decinormal or 0.1N or $\frac{N}{10}$ solution. The equivalent weight of potassium dichromate is 49.03. Substances whose standard solutions are prepared like this are known as main or primary standards.

However all substances cannot be used as primary standards. For any substance to be used as a primary standard, it must be highly pure to the extent of nearly 100% and also quite stable. It should not deteriorate during storage or be affected by exposure to atmosphere, that is, it should not be hygroscopic or deliquescent. Nor should it be affected by the oxygen or carbon dioxide of the atmosphere. It should not also change its composition through efflorescence and loss of water of hydration or through absorption of water. Only substances which satisfy these requirements can be used as primary standards and their solution may be prepared by accurate weighing of the required quantity of the substance and dissolving in water to produce the required volume of the solution accurately. For this purpose the substances are dissolved and made up to volume in standard or volumetric flasks which have been accurately calibrated.

Examples of primary standards are oxalic acid, potassium dichromate, sodium chloride, succinic acid, anhydrous sodium carbonate etc. The primary standard should be of analytical regent grade that is A.R. or G.R. (Guaranteed Reagent) quality supplied by reputed manufacturers.

In the case of anhydrous sodium carbonate, it is necessary to know that it absorbs water from the atmosphere when exposed and forms a mixture of hydrates. Solutions prepared out of such a substance will have a different normality other than what is calculated. Therefore the bottle containing anhydrous sodium carbonate should be kept tightly closed. In addition before every use it may be heated in a nickel crucible strongly to expel all the moisture and cooled in a desiccator.

In the second method the normality of a solution can be found out by titrating against a primary standard or a secondary standard. A secondary standard is a solution whose normality is already known by titrating against a primary standard. Standardization is the determination of the exact normality or molarity of a solution.

Thus a solution of sodium hydroxide may be standardized by titrating against a standard solution of oxalic acid (primary standard) or against a standard solution of hydrochloric acid (secondary standard).

A secondary standard is a substance which for one or more of the reasons already mentioned while dealing with primary standards cannot be used as a primary standard. For example, sodium hydroxide cannot be used as a primary standard for the reason that it absorbs water and carbon dioxide from the atmosphere and the composition of its solution is subject to wide variation at different periods. Similarly sodium thiosulphate absorbs carbon dioxide from the atmosphere and is decomposed. A deposit of sulphur settles at the bottom. Similarly the compositions of solutions of various other substances like mineral acids, potassium permanganate, iodine etc. are also variable at different times. Therefore these cannot be used as primary standards. The normality of the solution of such a substance can be found out by titrating against a standard solution of primary standard or in other words the solution may be standardized by titrating against the standard solution of a primary standard.

Titrations: Titration is the process in which a standard solution is added in a controlled manner to the solution of the substance which is estimated. The titrant is taken in the burette and the solution of the substance being estimated is taken in a conical or Erlenmeyer flask or vice versa. A suitable indicator is added to the solution in the conical flask. The titrant reacts with the substance being estimated. The end point is the point at which the titrant has just completely reacted with the substance in chemically equivalent quantity. To determine the end point a suitable indicator is used. Sometimes as in the case of potassium permanganate the titrant itself may act as a self indicator so that the next drop added after the end point is reached makes the solution in the conical flask faintly pink.

Indicators: Indicators are mainly used in acidimetry and alkalimetry and in some other titrations. They are able to change colour at different pH. When there is a sharp pH change at the end point, it is indicated by the indicator changing colour which enables one to stop the titration at this point.

The indicator for a particular titration must be correctly and carefully chosen. Thus methyl orange is preferably used in a titration between a strong acid and a strong base since the colour change at the end point is sharp and clear. However phenolphthalein or methyl red can also be used in this titration. Methyl orange is also used as the indicator in the titration of a weak base like sodium carbonate against a strong acid and phenolphthalein is used in the titration of a weak acid against a strong base.

Other indicators like potassium chromate or ferric ammonium sulphate are chemicals which react with the titrant to give permanent coloured precipitates (red) at the end point. There are also flourescent indicators which flouresce at the end point. Starch mucilage gives a blue colour with iodine which is discharged at the end point when the iodine solution is titrated with sodium thiosulphate solution.

The following are the pH ranges and colour changes of some of the common indicators:

Indicators	pH Range	Colour Change
Methyl orange	2.9 to 4.0	Red to yellow
Methyl red	4.2 to 6.3	Red to yellow
Bromothymol blue	6.0 to 7.6	Yellow to blue
Phenol red	6.8 to 8.4	Yellow to red
Thymol blue	8.0 to 9.6	Yellow to blue
Phenolphthalein	8.3 to 10.6	Colourless to red

Preparation of a Volumetric Solution and its Standardization

As already stated, the standard solution of a primary standard like anhydrous sodium carbonate is prepared by weighing the required quantity of the substance and dissolving in the required quantity of water. For example for preparing 250 ml of a 1N solution of sodium carbonate, about 13.25 grams of sodium carbonate are actually weighed. It is transferred to a 250 ml volumetric or standard flask, distilled water is added to dissolve it and more distilled water is added to make up to volume. The flask is stoppered and shaken to ensure uniform mixing. Suppose the weight of anhydrous sodium carbonate taken is 13.5500 grams. The normality of the solution is calculated as below:

Equivalent weight of anhydrous sodium carbonate = 53.

53 grams in 1 litre of the solution will give a $\frac{N}{1}$ solution. But the volume in the present case is 250 ml. Therefore, $\frac{53}{4} = 13.25$ grams of anhydrous sodium carbonate are sufficient to give the $\frac{N}{1}$ solution. However the quantity weighted out is 13.5500 grams and not 13.25 grams. Therefore, eventhough it is a $\frac{N}{1}$ solution, yet its normality is not exactly $1.000\frac{N}{1}$.

Normality of the solution $= \frac{13.55}{13.25} = 1.023 \ \frac{N}{1}$. If a quantity less than 13.25 grams has been weighed out, then the normality will be less than $1.000 \ \frac{N}{1}$. Suppose only 13.0280 grams have been weighed, the normality will be

$$\frac{13.0280}{13.25} = 0.9833 \ \frac{N}{1}.$$

Similarly a decinormal solution of sodium carbonate may be prepared by taking accurately about one-tenth of the quantity required for preparing a normal solution and calculating its normality in the same way. Therefore the exact normality of solution is calculated by using the formula:

$$\text{Normality} = \frac{\textbf{Weight taken}}{\textbf{Weight to be taken}}$$

However the volumetric solution of a secondary standard is prepared by weighing the required quantity approximately and dissolving in the required volume of water. It is standardized by titrating an aliquot (a definite volume) against a standard solution of a suitable primary standard and calculating its normality from the titre value obtained.

For example, one litre of normal solution of sodium hydroxide is prepared by weighing approximately 40 grams (its gram - equivalent) and dissolving in water to make one litre.

Its normality may be found out by titrating against a standard solution of $\frac{N}{1}$ oxalic or succinic acid (primary standard). For this purpose 20 ml of oxalic acid solution is pipetted out into a clean conical flask, two or three drops of phenolphthalein solution are added as an indicator and titrated with the approximately normal solution of sodium hydroxide.

Let us assume that the titre-value is 21 ml and the normality of the oxalic acid solution is $1.002\frac{N}{1}$. To calculate the normality of sodium hydroxide solution, use the normality equation

$$V_1N_1 = V_2N_2$$

where V_1 = Volume of oxalic acid solution taken

N_1 = Normality of oxalic acid solution

V_2 = Titre value obtained

N_2 = Normality of sodium hydroxide solution

Normality of sodium hydroxide solution $V_1N_1 = V_2N_2$

$$N_2 = \frac{V_1N_1}{V_2} = \frac{20 \times 1.002}{21} = 0.9911\frac{N}{1}$$

This solution can be used as a secondary standard for finding out the normality of any other secondary standard like hydrochloric acid or sulphuric acid solution. Therefore the normality of any volumetric solution can be determined by titration against a standard solution of a primary or against a standard solution of a secondary standard of equivalent normality. It is also essential to remember that the normality of a volumetric solution of a secondary standard should be determined at the time of its use. This is because, since the composition of the solution of the secondary standard is subject to variation at different periods, the normality determined at an earlier date will not be strictly valid or accurate at a later date.

Titrimetric Assays of Inorganic Compounds

The majority of the assays of inorganic compounds are titrimetric assays. They are assayed either by straight titrations with the titrant or by back titrations. Back titrations are used when the substance being assayed is either insoluble or volatile. In back titrations the titrant is added in known excess to the substance which reacts with it quantitatively. The excess of the titrant, that is, the unreacted portion of the titrant, is four ' out by titration with a suitable standard solution. From this the actual volume of the titrant which was consumed by the substance is found out. Examples in this category are the assays of calcium carbonate (insoluble) and strong ammonia solution (volatile).

1. Acidimetry and Alkalimetry

Acidimetry and alkalimetry are methods used for the assay of bases and acids respectively. The bases are assayed by titration with acids (acidimetry) and the acids are assayed by titration with alkalis (alkalimetry). During these titrations the acids and bases neutralise each other and so the reaction is known as a neutralisation reaction. Where possible a straight titration is done and back titration is used in other cases for the reasons stated earlier. The following are estimated by acidimetry:-

1. Sodium bicarbonate
2. Sodium carbonate
3. Strong ammonia solution.

Boric acid and ammonium chloride are assayed by alkalimetry.

Preparation of Approximately $\frac{N}{1}$ Sulphuric Acid Solution

Aim: To prepare approximately $\frac{N}{1}$ sulphuric acid solution.

Procedure: Concentrated sulphuric acid is about 36N. So it should be diluted to get an approximately $\frac{N}{1}$ solution.

Add slowly with stirring 30 ml of concentrated sulphuric acid to 1000 ml of distilled water and allow to cool to 25°C. Shake well.

Standardization of $\frac{N}{1}$ Sulphuric Acid.

Aim: To standardize the approximately 1N sulphuric acid solution.

Principle: The sulphuric acid solution is standardized by titrating against standard $\frac{N}{1}$ sodium carbonate which is a primary standard.

$$H_2SO_4 + Na_2CO_3 \longrightarrow Na_2SO_4 + CO_2\uparrow + H_2O$$

Procedure: Heat anhydrous sodium carbonate, A.R. at 270°C for one hour and cool in a desiccator. Weigh about 5.3 g accurately and transfer to a 100 ml volumetric flask. Add distilled water to dissolve and make upto volume with more distilled water. Stopper the flask and mix well.

Pipette out 20 ml of the sodium carbonate solution into a clean conical flask and add two drops of methyl orange indicator solution. Titrate with $\frac{N}{1}$ sulphuric acid taken in the burette. End point is the appearance of a faint red colour. Repeat the titration to get concordant values.

Calculation

Equivalent weight of anhydrous sodium carbonate = 53

53 gm —— 1000 ml —— $\frac{N}{1}$ solution.

5.3 g —— 100 ml —— $\frac{N}{1}$ solution.

Weight to be taken for 100 ml = 5.3 g.

Normality of $\frac{N}{1}$ sodium carbonate $= \dfrac{\text{Weight taken}}{\text{Weight to be taken}}$

$$= \dfrac{\text{Weight taken}}{5.3} = x\,\frac{N}{1}$$

Normality $\frac{N}{1}$ sulphuric acid $= V_1N_1 = V_2N_2$

$$= 20 \times x = \text{Titre value} \times N_2$$

$$N_2 = \dfrac{20 \times x}{\text{Titre Value}} = y\,\frac{N}{1}$$

Preparation of $\frac{N}{2}$ Sulphuric Acid

Aim: To prepare approximately $\frac{N}{2}$ sulphuric acid solution.

Procedure

1. Dilute 500 ml of $\frac{N}{1}$ Sulphuric acid to 1000 ml with distilled water.

2. Add slowly with stirring 15 ml of concentrated sulphuric acid to 1000 ml of distilled water and allow to cool to 25°C. Shake well.

Any one of the above methods can be employed.

Standardization of $\frac{N}{2}$ Sulphuric Acid

Aim: To standardize the approximately $\frac{N}{2}$ sulphuric acid solution.

Procedure:

1. Weigh about 2.65 g of anhydrous sodium carbonate, A.R.(previously heated and cooled), transfer to a 100 ml standard flask, add water to dissolve and make up to volume. Stopper the flask and shake well.

2. Pipette out 50 ml of standard $\frac{N}{1}$ sodium carbonate (prepared above) into a clean 100 ml standard flask and dilute with distilled water upto the mark. Stopper the flask and shake well.

Any one of the above methods can be employed. If No.(2) is employed, there is no need for calculating the normality of the $\frac{N}{2}$ sodium carbonate solution prepared. The normality of the $\frac{N}{1}$ sodium carbonate (x) can be taken as the normality of $\frac{N}{2}$ sodium carbonate also $(x\frac{N}{2})$.

Pipette out 20 ml of the standard sodium carbonate solution into a clean conical flask and add two drops of methyl orange indicator solution. Titrate with $\frac{N}{2}$ sulphuric acid taken in the burette. End point is the appearance of a pale red colour. Repeat the titration to get concordant values.

Calculation

Equivalent weight of sodium carbonate = 53.

$$53 \text{ g} \underline{\hspace{1cm}} 1000 \text{ ml} \underline{\hspace{1cm}} \frac{N}{1}$$

$$5.3 \text{ g} \underline{\hspace{1cm}} 100 \text{ ml} \underline{\hspace{1cm}} \frac{N}{1}$$

$$2.65 \text{ g} \underline{\hspace{1cm}} 100 \text{ ml} \underline{\hspace{1cm}} \frac{N}{2}$$

Calculation for the normality of $\frac{N}{2}$ sulphuric acid is the same as for the normality of $\frac{N}{1}$ sulphuric acid.

Preparation of $\frac{N}{1}$ Sodium Hydroxide Solution.

Aim: To prepare approximately $\frac{N}{1}$ sodium hydroxide solution.

Procedure: Since equivalent weight of sodium hydroxide is 40, weigh about 40 grams of sodium hydroxide and dissolve in enough carbon dioxide-free water to produce 1000 ml. Mix well. Keep the solution tightly closed to avoid absorption of carbon dioxide from the atmosphere.

Standardization of $\frac{N}{1}$ Sodium Hydroxide

Aim: To standardise the approximately $\frac{N}{1}$ sodium hydroxide solution.

Principle: First standard $\frac{N}{1}$ oxalic acid or succinic acid solution is prepared. It is titrated against the approximately $\frac{N}{1}$ sodium hydroxide solution. The normality of $\frac{N}{1}$ sodium hydroxide is calculated using the normality equation.

$$(COOH)_2 + 2\,NaOH \longrightarrow (COONa)_2 + 2H_2O$$

Procedure: Weigh about 6.3 g of oxalic acid, A.R. accurately and transfer to a clean 100 ml standard flask. Add enough distilled water to dissolve it and make up to the mark with more distilled water. Stopper the flask and shake well.

Pipette out 20 ml of the oxalic acid solution into a clean conical flask and add two drops of phenolphthalein indicator solution. Titrate with sodium hydroxide solution till a permanent faint pink colour appears. Repeat the titration to get concordant values.

Calculation: Equivalent weight of oxalic acid = 63

$$63 \text{ g} \text{----} 1000 \text{ ml} \text{----} \frac{N}{1}$$

$$6.3 \text{ g} \text{----} 100 \text{ ml} \text{----} \frac{N}{1}$$

$$\text{Normality of oxalic acid} = \frac{\text{Weight taken}}{\text{Weight to be taken}} = x\ \frac{N}{1}$$

$$\text{Normality of sodium hydroxide} = V_1 N_1 = V_2 N_2,$$
$$= 20 \times x = T \times N_2.$$

$$N_2 = \frac{20 \times x}{T} = y.$$

where x = normality of oxalic acid solution.
$\quad\ \ $ T = titre value
$\quad\ \ y$ = normality of sodium hydroxide solution.

1. Assay of Sodium Bicarbonate

Aim: To assay the given sample of sodium bicarbonate and calculate its percentage purity (% w/w).

Principle: Sodium bicarbonate in aqueous solution is titrated with $\frac{N}{1}$ sulphuric acid, using methyl orange as indicator.

$$2NaHCO_3 + H_2SO_4 \longrightarrow Na_2SO_4 + 2CO_2\uparrow + 2H_2O$$

Procedure: Weigh accurately about 1 g of the sample into a clean conical flask nd dissolve in 20 ml of water. Titrate with $\frac{N}{2}$ sulphuric acid, using methyl orange solution as indicator till a faint red colour appears. Each ml of $\frac{N}{1}$ sulphuric acid is equivalent to 0.042 g of $NaHCO_3$.

Calculation: % w/v of $NaHCO_3 = \dfrac{T \times N \times 0.042 \times 100}{\text{Weight taken}}$.

$\qquad$ T = titre value
$\qquad$ N = Normality of sulphuric acid.

In this calculation 0.042 g is known as the **factor**. It gives the amount of sodium bicarbonate which is equivalent to one ml of $\frac{N}{2}$ sulphuric acid. Since volumetric solutions of equal normality are supposed to be reacting in equal volumes, the amount of sodium bicarbonate present in the sample can be obtained by finding out the volume of $\frac{N}{2}$ sulphuric acid required to react with it and multiplying the same with the factor of sodium bicarbonate.

Calculation of Factor:

$\qquad$ Equivalent weight of sodium bicarbonate = 84. 84 grams in one litre of the solution give a 1 N or $\frac{N}{1}$ solution.

$$\text{or} \quad 84\ g \text{——} 1000\ ml \text{——} \frac{N}{1}$$
$$42\ g \text{——} 1000\ ml \text{——} \frac{N}{2}$$
$$0.042\ g\ \left(\frac{42}{1000}\right) \text{——} 1\ ml \text{——} \frac{N}{2}$$

$\qquad$ Therefore each ml of $\frac{N}{2}$ sulphuric acid is equivalent to 0.042 g of $NaHCO_3$.

Assay of Sodium Bicarbonate Solution

Aim: To assay the given sodium bicarbonate solution and calculate the amount of sodium bicarbonate present in 100 ml of the solution (% w/v).

Principle: Same as for assay of sodium bicarbonate.

Procedure: Pipette out 20 ml of the solution into a clean conical flask, add two drops of methyl orange solution and titrate with standard $\frac{N}{2}$ sulphuric acid till the solution acquires a faint red colour. Repeat the titration to get concordant values. Each ml of $\frac{N}{2}$ sulphuric acid is equivalent to to 0.042 g of $NaHCO_3$.

Calculation

$$\text{Amount of sodium bicarbon present in 100 ml of the solution} = \frac{T \times N \times 0.042 \times 100}{\text{Volume taken}}$$

or

$$\%\ \text{w/v of NaHCO3} = \frac{T \times N \times 0.042 \times 100}{20}$$

Note: Sodium bicarbonate in solution slowly decomposes to form sodium carbonate, carbon dioxide and water.

If weight per litre is asked for, it can be calculated simply by multiplying by 1000 instead of by 100 as given below :

$$\frac{T \times N \times 0.042 \times 1000}{20}$$

2. Assay of Ammonia Solution Strong

Aim: To assay the given sample of Ammonia Solution Strong and calculate the amount of ammonia present in 100 g of the solution (% w/w).

Principle: Ammonia Solution Strong, being volatile, can be estimated only by back titration. So to the sample is added a known excess of $\frac{N}{1}$ sulphuric acid. The excess of sulphuric acid is back titrated with $\frac{N}{1}$ sodium hydroxide using methyl red solution as indicator. The reactions are as given below:

$$2NH_4OH + H_2SO_4 \longrightarrow (NH_4)_2\,SO_4 + 2H_2O$$

$$H_2SO_4 + 2NaOH \longrightarrow Na_2SO_4 + 2H_2O$$

Procedure: Weigh accurately about 3 g of the sample and transfer to a clean conical flask. Add exactly by pipetting 50 ml of standard $\frac{N}{1}$ sulphuric acid and titrate the excess of acid with standard $\frac{N}{1}$ sodium hydroxide using methyl red solution as indicator till a faint yellow colour appears. Each ml of $\frac{N}{1}$ sodium hydroxide is equivalent to 0.01703 g of NH_3.

Calculation

Amount of ammonia present in 100 g of the solution or % w/w of NH_3 $= \dfrac{(50 \times N_1) - (T \times N_2) \times 0.01703 \times 100}{\text{Weight taken}}$

$$N_1 = \text{Normality of acid}$$
$$T = \text{Titre value}$$
$$N_2 = \text{Normality of alkali.}$$

Calculation of Factor:

Equivalent weight of ammonia = 17.03

17.03 g —— 1000 ml —— $\frac{N}{1}$

0.01703 g —— 1 ml —— $\frac{N}{1}$

3. Assay of Boric Acid

Aim: To assay the given sample of boric acid and calculate its percentage purity.

Principle: Since boric acid is a weak tribasic acid, it cannot be titrated directly with sodium hydroxide solution. So neutralised glycerin is added to convert the boric acid into a stronger monobasic acid which can be titrated directly with sodium hydroxide solution. The reaction as given below:

$$2\ \begin{array}{c} CH_2OH \\ | \\ CHOH \\ | \\ CH_2OH \end{array} \ + \ \begin{array}{c} HO \\ \diagdown \\ HO-B \\ \diagup \\ HO \end{array} \rightarrow \left[\begin{array}{cc} H_2COH & HOCH_2 \\ | & | \\ HC-O & O-CH \\ & \diagdown \ B \ \diagup & \\ | & | \\ H_2C-O & O-CH_2 \end{array} \right]^{-}$$

Procedure: Weigh accurately about 2 g of the sample. Dissolve it in a mixture of 50 ml of water and 100 ml of glycerin (previously neutralised to phenolphthalein) in a clean conical flask. Titrate with $\frac{N}{1}$ sodium hydroxide using phenolphthalein solution as indicator till a faint permanent pink colour appears in the solution. Each ml of $\frac{N}{1}$ sodium hydroxide is equivalent to 0.06183 g. of H_3BO_3.

Calculation:

$$\% \text{ w/w of boric acid} = \frac{T \times N \times 0.06183 \times 100}{\text{Weight taken}}$$

Calculation of Factor:

Equivalent weight of boric acid = 61.83 g.

$$61.83 \text{ g} \text{———} 1000 \text{ ml} \text{———} \frac{N}{1}$$
$$0.06183 \text{ g} \text{———} 1 \text{ ml} \text{———} \frac{N}{1}$$

Assay of Boric Acid Solution

Aim: to assay the given boric acid solution and calculate the amount present in 100 ml of the solution (% w/v).

Principle: Same as for the Assay of Boric Acid.

Procedure: Pipette out 20 ml of the given boric acid solution into a clean conical flask and add 10 ml of glycerol previously neutralised to phenolphthalein. Titrate with standard $\frac{N}{10}$ sodium hydroxide solution using phenolphthalein solution as indicator till a faint permanent pink colour appears. Repeat the titration to get concordant values. Each ml of sodium hydroxide is equivalent to 0.006183 g of boric acid.

Calculation of Factor

$$0.06183 \text{ g} \longrightarrow 1 \text{ ml} \longrightarrow \frac{N}{1}$$

$$0.006183 \text{ g} \longrightarrow 1 \text{ ml} \longrightarrow \frac{N}{10}$$

Note: The decinormal sodium hydroxide solution required for this assay may be prepared by diluting $\frac{N}{1}$ sodium hydroxide ten times and standardized by titrating with standard decinormal oxalic acid.

4. Assay of Ammonium Chloride (I.P.1985)

Aim: To assay the given sample of ammonium chloride and calculate its percentage purity.

Principle: To a solution of ammonium chloride in water is added neutralised and diluted formaldehyde solution. Formaldehyde converts the ammonium part into hexamine. An equivalent quantity of hydrochloric acid is liberated.

$$4 \text{ NH}_4\text{Cl} + 6\text{HCHO} \longrightarrow (\text{CH}_2)_6\text{N}_4 + 4 \text{ HCl} + 6 \text{ H}_2\text{O}$$

        Formaldehyde   Hexamine

The acid is titrated with standard alkali using phenolphthalein solution as indicator. Care is taken to ensure that the formaldehyde solution is strictly neutral (by neutralising it with very dilute alkali using phenolphthalein as indicator) and does not add to the acidity in the solution.

Procedure: Weigh accurately about 0.1 g of ammonium chloride and transfer to a clean conical flask. Dissolve in 20 ml of water. Add a mixture of 5 ml of formaldehyde, previously neutralised to phenolphthalein and 20 ml of water. Allow to stand for 10 minutes. Then titrate slowly with $\frac{N}{10}$ sodium hydroxide solution using phenolphthalein solution as indicator until a permanent pale pink colour appears. Each ml of $\frac{N}{10}$ sodium hydroxide is equivalent to 0.005349 g of NH_4Cl.

Calculation

$$\% \text{ w/w of ammonium chloride} = \frac{T \times N \times 0.005349 \times 100}{\text{Weight taken}}$$

Calculation of Factor

Equivalent weight of ammonium chloride = 53.49

$$53.49 \text{ g} \longrightarrow 1000 \text{ ml} \longrightarrow \frac{N}{1}$$

$$5.349 \text{ g} \longrightarrow 1000 \text{ ml} \longrightarrow \frac{N}{10}$$

$$0.005349 \text{ g} \longrightarrow 1 \text{ ml} \longrightarrow \frac{N}{10}$$

Assay of Ammonium Chloride Solution

Aim: To assay the given ammonium chloride solution and calculate the amount present in 100 ml of the solution (% w/v).

Principle: Same as for assay of ammonium chloride solution.

Procedure: Pipette out 20 ml of the given ammonium chloride solution into a clean conical flask. Add 5 ml of formaldehyde previously neutralised to phenolphthalein. Allow to stand for 10 minutes. Then titrate slowly with $\frac{N}{10}$ sodium hydroxide using phenolphthalein as indicator until a pale permanent pink colour appears. Repeat the titration get concordant values. Each ml of $\frac{N}{10}$ sodium hydroxide is equivalent to 0.005349 g of NH_4Cl.

Calculation:

$$\% \text{ w/v of ammonium chloride} = \frac{T \times N \times 0.005349 \times 100}{20}$$

Note: Ammonium chloride is assayed by an argentimetric method in I.P. '66.

Oxidation - Reduction

An oxidizing agent oxidises reducing agents, itself getting reduced in the process. So oxidising and reducing agents can be used for the standardization and estimation of each other.

The oxidising agents in common use in analytical chemistry are potassium permanganate, potassium dichromate, ceric sulphate, iodine etc. The reducing agents are oxalic acid, sodium oxalate, ferrous sulphate, sodium thiosulphate etc.

II. Permanganimetry

In permanganimetry decinormal solution of potassium permanganate is used. Many substances which are oxidized by potassium permanganate are assayed by titration against standard $\frac{N}{10}$ potassium permanganate.

As already stated in Theory, potassium permanganate evolves nascent oxygen in acid or alkaline solution which is responsible for the oxidation.

$$2KMnO_4 + 3H_2SO_4 \longrightarrow K_2SO_4 + 2MnSO_4 + 3H_2O + 5(O)$$
$$\text{(acid solution)}$$

$$2\ KMnO_4 + H_2O \longrightarrow 2MnO_2 + 2KOH + 3(O)$$
$$\text{(alkaline or neutral solution)}$$

Decinormal potassium permanganate solution is standardized by titration against a primary standard like sodium oxalate, oxalic acid, ferrous sulphate etc. The potassium permanganate is always taken in the burette as the titrant and acts as a self-indicator, the end point being the appearance of a permanent faint pink colour.

Preparation of Approximately $\frac{N}{10}$ Potassium Permanganate

Aim: To prepare approximately $\frac{N}{10}$ potassium permanganate solution.

Procedure: Weigh about 3.3 g of potassium permanganate and dissolve in 1000 ml of water. Heat on a water bath for one hour and allow to stand for two days. Filter.

Calculation

Equivalent weight of potassium permanganate = 31.61

$$31.61 \text{ g} \longrightarrow 1000 \text{ ml} \longrightarrow \frac{N}{1}$$

$$3.161 \text{ g} \longrightarrow 1000 \text{ ml} \longrightarrow \frac{N}{10}$$

Standardization of $\frac{N}{10}$ Potassium Permanganate

Aim: To standardize the approximately $\frac{N}{10}$ potassium permanganate solution.

Principle: Potassium permanganate solution is standardized by titration against standard oxalic acid solution. Oxalic acid in the presence of dilute sulphuric acid is oxidized by potassium permanganate to carbon dioxide and water. The oxalic acid solution should be warmed to $70^{\circ}C$ before the titration, as otherwise the reaction is slow.

$$5 \begin{array}{c} COOH \\ | \\ COOH \end{array} + 3H_2SO_4 + 2KMnO_4 \rightarrow K_2SO_4 + 2MnSO_4 + 8H_2O + 10CO_2\uparrow$$

$$\text{or } \begin{array}{c} COOH \\ | \\ COOH \end{array} + O \rightarrow 2CO_2\uparrow + H_2O$$

Procedure: Weigh exactly about 0.63 g of oxalic acid, A.R. and transfer to a 100 ml standard flask. Add enough water to dissolve and make up to the mark. Stopper the flask and shake well.

Pipette out 20 ml of the standard oxalic acid solution into a clean conical flask and add 20 ml of dilute sulphuric acid. Warm this solution to $70^{\circ}C$ and titrate with $\frac{N}{10}$ potassium permanganate till a permanent faint pink colour appears. Repeat the titration to get concordant values.

Calculation: First the normality of $\frac{N}{10}$ oxalic acid is calculated.

$$\text{Normality of oxalic acid} = \frac{\text{Weight taken}}{0.63}$$

Equivalent weight of oxalic acid = 63

$$63 \text{ g} \longrightarrow 1000 \text{ ml} \longrightarrow \frac{N}{1}$$

$$6.3 \text{ g} \longrightarrow 1000 \text{ ml} \longrightarrow \frac{N}{10}$$

$$0.63 \text{ g} \longrightarrow 100 \text{ ml} \longrightarrow \frac{N}{10}$$

Making use of the normality of oxalic acid solution, the normality of $\frac{N}{10}$ potassium permanganate is calculated by using the normality equation $V_1N_1 = V_2N_2$.

5. Assay of Hydrogen Peroxide Solution

Aim: To assay the given hydrogen peroxide solution and calculate the percentage weight in volume (%w/v) of hydrogen peroxide in the solution.

Principle: A mixture of hydrogen peroxide solution and dilute sulphuric acid is titrated against $\frac{N}{10}$ potassium permanganate. Hydrogen peroxide is oxidized by potassium permanganate to water and oxygen. Potassium permanganate acts as a self-indicator.

$$2 \text{ KMnO}_4 + 3H_2SO_4 + 5 \text{ H}_2O_2 \longrightarrow K_2SO_4 + 2MnSO_4$$
$$+ 8H_2O + 5O_2\uparrow$$

or $H_2O_2 + O \longrightarrow H_2O + O_2\uparrow$

Procedure: Pipette out 10 ml of the given hydrogen peroxide solution into a clean 250 ml volumetric flask. Make up to the mark with distilled water. Stopper the flask and shake well.

Pipette out 25 ml of this solution into a conical flask and add 5 ml of 5N sulphuric acid. Titrate with standard $\frac{N}{10}$ potassium permanganate till a permanent pale pink colour appears. Repeat the titration to get concordant values. Each ml of $\frac{N}{10}$ potassium permanganate is equivalent to 0.001701 g of H_2O_2.

Calculation

$$\% \text{ w/v of hydrogen peroxide} = \frac{T \times N \times 0.001701 \times 250 \times 10}{25}.$$

Initially the amount present in 250 ml of the diluted solution is calculated. Since the same amount is present in 10 ml of the undiluted solution, the % w/v of hydrogen peroxide is obtained by multiplying by 10.

Calculation of Factor

Equivalent weight of hydrogen peroxide = 17.01

$$17.01 \text{ g} \text{---} 1000 \text{ ml} \text{---} \frac{N}{1}$$

$$1.701 \text{ g} \text{---} 1000 \text{ ml} \text{---} \frac{N}{10}$$

$$0.001701 \text{ g} \text{---} 1 \text{ ml} \text{---} \frac{N}{10}$$

6. Assay of Ferrous Sulphate

Aim: To assay the given sample of ferrous sulphate and calculate its percentage purity (% w/w).

Principle: Ferrous sulphate solution is mixed with dilute sulphuric acid and titrated against standard $\frac{N}{10}$ potassium permanganate. Ferrous sulphate is oxidized to ferric sulphate by potassium permanganate which acts as a self indicator.

$$10FeSO_4 + 2KMnO_4 + 8H_2SO_4 \longrightarrow 5Fe_2(SO_4)_3$$
$$+ 2MnSO_4 + K_2SO_4 + 8H_2O$$

$$\text{or } 2FeSO_4 + H_2SO_4 + O \longrightarrow Fe_2(SO_4)_3 + H_2O$$

Procedure: Weigh accurately about 1 g of the sample of ferrous sulphate and dissolve in 20 ml of dilute sulphuric acid in a clean conical flask. Titrate with standard $\frac{N}{10}$ potassium permanganate till a permanent pale pink colour appears. Each ml of $\frac{N}{10}$ potassium permanganate is equivalent to 0.0278 g of $FeSO_4.7H_2O$.

Calculation: % w/w of ferrous sulphate $= \dfrac{T \times N \times 0.0278 \times 100}{\text{Weight taken}}$

Calculation of Factor

Equivalent weight of ferrous sulphate $= 278$

$$278 \text{ g} \text{---} 1000 \text{ ml} \text{---} \frac{N}{1}$$

$$27.8 \text{ g} \text{---} 1000 \text{ ml} \text{---} \frac{N}{10}$$

$$0.0278 \text{ g} \text{---} 1 \text{ ml} \text{---} \frac{N}{10}$$

Assay of Ferrous Sulphate Solution

Aim: To assay the given ferrous sulphate solution and calculate the 'percentage weight in volume (% w/v) of ferrous sulphate in the solution.

Principle: Same as for assay of ferrous sulphate.

Procedure: Pipette out 20 ml of the given ferrous sulphate solution into a clean conical flask and add 20 ml of dilute sulphuric acid. Titrate with standard $\frac{N}{10}$ potassium permanganate till the appearance of a permanent pale pink colour. Repeat the titration to get concordant values. Each ml of $\frac{N}{10}$ potassium permanganate is equivalent to 0.0278 g of $FeSO_4 \cdot 7H_2O$.

Calculation: % w/v of ferrous sulphate $= \dfrac{T \times N \times 0.0278 \times 100}{20}$

III. Iodimetry and Iodometry

In **iodimetry** a standard solution of iodine is used for assaying reducing agents like ascorbic acid. In **iodometry** iodine is liberated from potassium iodide by an oxidizing agent and this iodine is titrated against standard sodium thiosulphate solution. By this way many compounds like copper sulphate and chlorinated lime are assayed.

Sodium thiosulphate ($Na_2S_2O_3 \cdot 5H_2O$) cannot be used as a primary standard for the reason that it is efflorescent and so its composition is variable. Secondly, as already stated it precipitates sulphur on absorbing carbon dioxide from the atmosphere. Therefore an approximately decinormal solution is prepared and standardized before use by titration against standard $\frac{N}{10}$ potassium dichromate.

Preparation of $\frac{N}{10}$ Sodium Thiosulphate

Aim: To prepare approximately decinormal sodium thiosulphate solution.

Procedure: Weigh about 26 g of sodium thiosulphate and 0.2 g of sodium carbonate and dissolve in carbon dioxide-free water. Add more of the same solvent to produce 1000 ml.

Sodium carbonate is added to give a pH of about 9.5 to the sodium thiosulphate solution. This pH discourages any bacterial action in the sodium thiosulphate which will be decomposed by the bacterial action. Use of carbon dioxide-free water is also necessary for the same reason. It may be prepared by boiling distilled water and cooling in a closed container to prevent reabsorption of carbon dioxide.

Calculation:

Equivalent weight of sodium thiosulphate = 248.2

$$248.2 \text{ g} \text{------} 1000 \text{ ml} \text{------} \frac{N}{1}$$

$$24.82 \text{ g} \text{------} 1000 \text{ ml} \text{------} \frac{N}{10}$$

Standardization of $\frac{N}{10}$ Sodium Thiosulphate Solution.

Aim: To standardize the approximately decinormal sodium thiosulphate solution.

Principle: Standard $\frac{N}{10}$ potassium dichromate solution is prepared. To an aliquot of this are added a mineral acid and potassium iodide. Iodine is liberated due to the oxidation of potassium iodide by the dichromate.

$$K_2Cr_2O_7 + 8 \text{ HCl} \longrightarrow 2 \text{ KCl} + 2CrCl_3 + 4H_2O + 3(O)$$

$$KI + HCl \longrightarrow KCl + HI$$

$$2HI + O \longrightarrow H_2O + I_2$$

The liberated iodine is titrated against $\frac{N}{10}$ sodium thiosulphate solution, using starch mucilage as indicator towards the end of the titration. End point is the disappearance of the blue colour and the appearance of the green colour.

$$I_2 + 2Na_2S_2O_3 \longrightarrow Na_2S_4O_6 + 2NaI$$

Procedure: Weigh about 0.4903 g of potassium dichromate, A.R. accurately and transfer to a clean 100 ml standard flask. Add enough distilled water to dissolve and make up to the mark with more distilled water. Stopper the flask and shake well.

Pipette out 20 ml of the potassium dichromate solution into a clean conical flask and add 5 ml of concentrated hydrochloric acid and 10 ml of 20% w/v solution of potassium iodide. Titrate the liberated iodine with $\frac{N}{10}$ sodium thiosulphate solution till a straw yellow colour is obtained. Add 1 ml of starch mucilage as indicator and continue the titration till the blue colour just disappears and a green colour appears. Repeat the titration to get concordant values.

Calculation:

Equivalent weight of potassium dichromate = 49.03

$$49.03\ g \text{——} 1000\ ml \text{——} \frac{N}{1}$$

$$4.903\ g \text{——} 1000\ ml \text{——} \frac{N}{10}$$

$$0.4903\ g \text{——} 100\ ml \text{——} \frac{N}{10}$$

Calculate the normality of $\frac{N}{10}$ sodium thiosulphate by using the normality equation $V_1N_1 = V_2N_2$.

7. Assay of Iodine Solution (Weak and Strong)

Aim: To assay the weak iodine solution for its content of iodine (% w/v).

Principle: Iodine in the solution is titrated with sodium thiosulphate solution which reduces it. Starch mucilage is used as the indicator towards the end of the titration when the solution has a straw yellow colour.

243

$$I_2 + 2Na_2S_2O_3 \longrightarrow Na_2S_4O_6 + 2\,NaI$$

End point is the disappearance of blue colour.

Procedure: Pipette out 10 ml of the weak iodine solution into a clean conical flask and add 20 ml of water. Titrate with standard $\frac{N}{10}$ sodium thiosulphate solution till the solution in the conical flask is straw yellow in colour. Add 1 ml of starch mucilage and titrate till the blue colour is discharged. Repeat the titration to get concordant values. Each ml of $\frac{N}{10}$ sodium thiosulphate is equivalent to 0.01269 g of I.

Calculation

$$\% \text{ w/v of I} = \frac{T \times N \times 0.01269 \times 100}{10}$$

Calculation of Factor

Equivalent weight of iodine $= 126.9$

$$126.9 \text{ g} \longrightarrow 1000 \text{ ml} \longrightarrow \frac{N}{1}$$

$$12.69 \text{ g} \longrightarrow 1000 \text{ ml} \longrightarrow \frac{N}{10}$$

$$0.01269 \text{ g} \longrightarrow 1 \text{ ml} \longrightarrow \frac{N}{10}$$

8. Assay of Chlorinated Lime (I.P.66)

Aim: To assay the given sample of chlorinated lime and calculate its content of available chlorine in terms of percentage weight in weight (% w/w).

Principle: When acetic acid and potassium iodide are added to a suspension of chlorinated lime in water, iodine is liberated. The chlorine present in the chlorinated lime replaces and liberates the iodine from potassium iodide.

$$CaCl(OCl) + 2CH_3COOH \longrightarrow (CH_3COO)_2\,Ca + HCl + HOCl$$

$$HCl + HOCl \longrightarrow Cl_2 + H_2O.$$

$$KI + CH_3COOH \longrightarrow CH_3COOK + HI$$

244

$$2HI + Cl_2 \longrightarrow I_2 + 2\,HCl$$

The liberated iodine is titrated with $\frac{N}{10}$ sodium thiosulphate solution.

$$I_2 + 2Na_2S_2O_3 \longrightarrow Na_2S_4O_6 + 2NaI$$

Starch mucilage is used as the indicator.

Procedure: Weigh about 4 g of the sample accurately and triturate in a mortar with successive small quantities of water. Transfer to an 1 litre standard flask and dilute to the mark. Stopper the flask and shake well.

Pipette out 100 ml of this suspension into a clean conical flask and add 3 g of potassium iodide and 5 ml of acetic acid.

Titrate the liberated iodine with $\frac{N}{10}$ sodium thiosulphate solution till it becomes straw yellow in colour. Add 1 ml of starch mucilage and continue the titration till the blue colour is discharged. Each ml of $\frac{N}{10}$ sodium thiosulphate is equivalent to 0.003545 g of available chlorine.

Calculation

$$\text{\% w/v of available chlorine} = \frac{T \times N \times 0.003545 \times 10 \times 100}{\text{Weight taken}}$$

The weight taken is made into a suspension of 1000 ml. Only 100 ml of this is taken for the assay. So the assay is for 100 ml of the solution only. Multiply by 10 to get the value for 1000 ml which contains the weight taken. Find out the percentage w/v of available chlorine by multiplying by 100 and dividing by the weight taken.

Calculation of Factor

The assay is to find out the content of available chlorine in the sample of chlorinated lime.

Equivalent weight of chlorine = 35.45

$$35.45 \text{ g} \text{——} 1000 \text{ ml} \text{——} \frac{N}{1}$$

$$3.545 \text{ g} \text{——} 1000 \text{ ml} \text{——} \frac{N}{10}$$

$$0.003545 \text{ g} \text{——} 1 \text{ ml} \text{——} \frac{N}{10}$$

V. Argentimetry

Argentimetry involves the use of a standard solution of silver nitrate as the titrant for the estimation of halides, that is, chlorides, bromides and iodides. For this a decinormal solution of silver nitrate should be prepared. Two methods can be used for this. Silver nitrate, A.R. is 99.9 percent pure. It can be treated as a primary standard and about one-tenth of its gram-equivalent weight, accurately weighed, may be dissolved in water to produce 1000 ml to give a decinormal solution. In the other method an approximately decinormal solution is prepared just as in the case if any secondary standard by weighing out an approximate quantity of silver nitrate and dissolving in distilled water and making up to volume approximately. It can be standardized by titration against a standard decinormal solution of sodium chloride which is a primary standard. Silver nitrate is photosensitive (affected by light) and so its solution should be stored in an amber glass bottle.

The halides are estimated by titration against silver nitrate in two ways:

1. Mohr's method: In this method, the neutral solution of the halide is titrated against standard decinormal silver nitrate. Potassium chromate solution is used as the indicator. After all the halide has been precipitated as silver halide, the next drop of silver nitrate combines with the potassium chromate to produce silver chromate which is red in colour. This is the end point. Sodium chloride can be estimated like this.

2. Volhard's method: Mohr's method cannot be used in acid solution but only neutral solution. So if the solution to be titrated is acid, Mohr's method is ruled out. This is because the silver chromate formed at the end point is soluble in acid. In such cases Vohard's method can be used.

In this method a known excess of standard silver nitrate solution is added to the chloride solution in the conical flask. Silver chloride is precipitated as a curdy, white precipitate. The excess of silver nitrate is titrated against standard decinormal ammonium thiocyanate. Ferric ammonium sulphate (ferric alum) is used as the indicator. Appearance of a permanent red colour is the end point. However in the case of a chloride it is necessary to filter off the silver chloride precipitate before titration with ammonium thiocyanate. Alternatively, the precipitate of

246

silver chloride may be coagulated by the addition of nitrobenzene before the titration. This is because silver chloride tends to react slowly with ammonium thiocyanate.

These titrations are also known as precipitation titrations since silver halide is precipitated.

Sodium chloride, its solutions and its injection were assayed (in I.P.65) by Mohr's method. However I.P.1985 has given Volhard's method for the assay. In this method sodium chloride is assayed by the addition of silver nitrate and the subsequent back titration of excess silver nitrate with ammonium thiocyanate in the presence of nitric acid.

Ammonium chloride was previously (I.P.66) assayed by Volhard's method. Now the assay in I.P.85 is different and is an alkalimetry method. Refer under Acidimetry and Alkalimetry.

Preparation of $\frac{N}{10}$ Silver Nitrate Solution

Aim: To prepare approximately decinormal silver nitrate solution.

Procedure: Weigh about 18 grams of silver nitrate and dissolve in sufficient volume of distilled water. Add more distilled water to produce 1000 ml. Store the solution in an amber glass bottle.

Calculation: Equivalent weight of silver nitrate $=$ 169.89

$$169.89 \text{ g} \longrightarrow 1000 \text{ ml} \longrightarrow \frac{N}{1}$$

$$16.989 \text{ g} \longrightarrow 1000 \text{ ml} \longrightarrow \frac{N}{10}$$

Standardization of $\frac{N}{10}$ Silver Nitrate Solution

Aim: To standardize the approximately decinormal silver nitrate solution.

Principle: The decinormal solution of silver nitrate is standardized by titration against standard decinormal solution of sodium chloride which is a primary standard. Therefore first standard decinormal solution of sodium chloride is prepared and it is used for standardizing the approximately decinormal solution of silver nitrate.

$$\text{Ag NO}_3 + \text{NaCl} \longrightarrow \text{AgCl}\downarrow + \text{NaNO}_3$$

Procedure: Weigh accurately about 0.5845 g of sodium chloride, A.R. and transfer to a 100 ml volumetric flask. Add sufficient quantity of distilled water to dissolve. Make up to the mark by adding more distilled water. Stopper the flask and shake well.

Pipette out 20 ml of the sodium chloride solution into a clean conical flask. Add 1 ml of potassium chromate solution. Titrate with the decinormal silver nitrate solution till a permanent faint reddish brown colour appears. Repeat the titration to get concordant values.

Calculation: The amount of sodium chloride to be taken is calculated as follows:

Equivalent weight of sodium chloride = 58.45

$$58.45 \text{ g} \underline{\hspace{1cm}} 1000 \text{ ml} \underline{\hspace{1cm}} \frac{N}{1}$$

$$5.845 \text{ g} \underline{\hspace{1cm}} 1000 \text{ ml} \underline{\hspace{1cm}} \frac{N}{10}$$

$$0.5845 \text{ g} \underline{\hspace{1cm}} 100 \text{ ml} \underline{\hspace{1cm}} \frac{N}{10}$$

The normality of the sodium chloride solution is calculated by using the formula.

$$\frac{\text{Weight taken}}{\text{Weight to be taken}} = \frac{\text{Weight taken}}{0.5845}$$

Then using this, calculate the normality of the silver nitrate solution by the normality equation $V_1N_1 = V_2N_2$

Preparation of $\frac{N}{10}$ Ammonium Thiocyanate Solution

Aim: To prepare approximately decinormal ammonium thiocyanate solution.

Procedure : Weigh about 8 grams of ammonium thiocyanate and dissolve in sufficient quantity of water. Add more water to produce 1000 ml. Stopper and shake well.

Calculation

Equivalent weight of ammonium thiocyanate = 76.12

$$76.12 \text{ g} \underline{\hspace{1cm}} 1000 \text{ ml} \underline{\hspace{1cm}} \frac{N}{1}$$

$$7.612 \text{ g} \underline{\hspace{1cm}} 1000 \text{ ml} \underline{\hspace{1cm}} \frac{N}{10}$$

Since ammonium thiocynate is a deliquescent substance, it is treated as a secondary standard. For this reason also slightly more of the substance than what is required is taken to prepare the decinormal solution.

Standardization of $\frac{N}{10}$ Ammonium Thiocyanate Solution

Aim: To standardize the approximately decinormal ammonium thiocyanate solution.

Principle: Standard decinormal silver nitrate solution is mixed with nitric acid and titrated against the approximately decinormal ammonium thiocyanate solution. End point is the appearance of a faint reddish brown colour.

$$NH_4SCN + AgNO_3 \longrightarrow AgSCN + NH_4NO_3$$
Ammonium
thiocyanate

Procedure: Pipette out 20 ml of standard $\frac{N}{10}$ silver nitrate into a clean conical flask. Add 2 ml of concentrated nitric acid and 2 ml of ferric ammonium sulphate solution. Titrate with ammonium thiocyanate solution till a faint reddish brown colour appears. Repeat the titration to get concordant values.

Calculation: Using the normality of standard decinormal silver nitrate solution, calculate the normality of the $\frac{N}{10}$ ammonium thiocyanate solution by the normality equation $V_1N_1 = V_2N_2$.

9. Assay of Sodium Chloride Injection, I.P.

Aim: To assay the given sample of sodium chloride injection for its content of sodium chloride (% w/v).

Principle: This assay is done by Volhard's method. To the sodium chloride injection are added a known excess of silver nitrate solution, concentrated nitric acid and nitrobenzene. Silver chloride is precipitated.

$$AgNO_3 + NaCl \longrightarrow AgCl\downarrow + NaNO_3$$

Nitrobenzene coagulates the silver chloride precipitate. The excess of silver nitrate is titrated against standard $\frac{N}{10}$ ammonium thiocyanate, using ferric ammonium sulphate as indicator.

$$NH_4SCN + AgNO_3 \longrightarrow AgSCN + NH_4NO_3$$

Procedure: Pipette out 30 ml of the sodium chloride injection into a clean conical flask and add 20 ml of distilled water. Add 50 ml (by pipetting) of standard $\frac{N}{10}$ silver nitrate solution, 3 ml of concentrated nitric acid, 5 ml of nitrobenzene and 2 ml of ferric ammonium sulphate solution and shake. Titrate with standard $\frac{N}{10}$ ammonium thiocyanate solution until the appearance of a faint reddish brown colour Each ml of $\frac{N}{10}$ silver nitrate is equivalent to 0.005844 g of sodium chloride.

Calculation: This is a back titration. So the normalities of both silver nitrate and ammonium thiocyanate solutions should be known already.

$$\% \text{ w/v of NaCl} = \frac{(50 \times N_1) - (T \times N_2) \times 0.005844 \times 100}{30}$$

N_1 = Normality of silver nitrate solution

N_2 = Normality of ammonium thiocyanate solution

T = Titre value

Calculation of Factor:

Equivalent weight of sodium chloride = 58.44

$$58.44 \text{ g} \longrightarrow 1000 \text{ ml} \longrightarrow \frac{N}{1}$$

$$5.844 \text{ g} \longrightarrow 1000 \text{ ml} \longrightarrow \frac{N}{10}$$

$$0.005844 \text{ g} \longrightarrow 1 \text{ ml} \longrightarrow \frac{N}{10}$$

10. Assay of Ammonium Chloride (I.P.1966)

Aim: To assay the given sample of ammonium chloride and calculate

Principle: Ammonium chloride forms an acidic solution when dissolved in water. So it is assayed by Volhard's method. To an aqueous solution of the ammonium chloride are added nitric acid, nitrobenzene and a known excess of $\frac{N}{10}$ silver nitrate and shaken vigorously. Silver chloride is precipitated and it is coagulated by nitrobenzene. This is done to prevent the silver chloride from reacting with the ammonium thiocyanate in the subsequent titration.

$$NH_4Cl + AgNO_3 \longrightarrow AgCl\downarrow + NH_4NO_3$$

Finally it is titrated with $\frac{N}{10}$ ammonium thiocyanate, using ferric ammonium sulphate as indicator.

$$NH_4SCN + AgNO_3 \longrightarrow AgSCN + NH_4NO_3$$

Procedure: Weigh about 0.2 g of the sample accurately and transfer to a clean conical flask. Add 3 ml of concentrated nitric acid and 5 ml of nitrobenzene. Add 50 ml of standard $\frac{N}{10}$ silver nitrate solution (by pipetting) and shake vigorously for one minute. Titrate with standard $\frac{N}{10}$ ammonium thiocyanate, using ferric ammonium sulphate solution as indicator. Each ml of $\frac{N}{10}$ silver nitrate is equivalent to 0.005349 g of NH$_4$Cl.

Calculation: This is a back titration. So the normalities of both silver nitrate and ammonium thiocyanate solutions should be known already

$$\% \text{ w/v of NaCl} = \frac{(50 \times N_1) - (T \times N_2) \times 0.005349 \times 100}{\text{Weight taken}}$$

N_1 = Normality of silver nitrate solution

N_2 = Normality of ammonium thiocyanate solution

T = Titre value

Calculation of Factor:

Equivalent weight of sodium chloride $=$ 53.49

53.49 g —— 1000 ml —— $\frac{N}{1}$

5.349 g —— 1000 ml —— $\frac{N}{10}$

$$0.005349 \text{ g} \underline{\hspace{1cm}} 1 \text{ ml} \underline{\hspace{1cm}} \frac{N}{10}$$

Note: Ammonium chloride is assayed by an alkalimetry method in I.P.1985.

VI. Complexometry

Complexometry means estimation through complex formation. Metals are complexed by complexing agents. A water soluble complex or chelate is formed. The metal is now in an unionisable condition. E.D.T.A. which is the disodium salt of ethylene diaminetetraacetic acid or sodium edetate is conveniently used as the chelating agent because of certain advantages. Most of the calcium, magnesium and lead salts in the I.P. are assayed by complexometric titration with E.D.T.A.

Just as in any other volumetric titration visual indicators are used in complexometric titrations also. They are known as metallochrome indicators. These indicators are themselves complexing agents which combine with the metal. When combined with the metal, the indicator has a particular colour. The metal is released by the indicator to the E.D.T.A. at the end point. The indicator is now in the free state and resumes its original colour. For example Eriochrome Black T is a metallochrome indicator with a natural blue colour. When combined with magnesium, the resulting complex has a wine red colour. At the end point the metal is taken away from the indicator by the E.D.T.A. and the indicator, being now in the free state, gets back its original blue colour. Therefore the end point in this titration is marked by a change of colour from wine red to blue. Eriochrome Black T is also known as Solochrome Black T or mordant black.

M/20 E.D.T.A. solution is prepared approximately and standardized by titration against solution of calcium carbonate, A.R.

11. Assay of Magnesium Sulphate (I.P.1985)

Aim: To assay the given sample of magnesium sulphate and calculate its percentage purity.

Principle: Magnesium sulphate is dissolved in water and titrated against M/20 E.D.T.A. solution. During the titration with E.D.T.A. magnesium is complexed and E.D.T.A.–magnesium complex is formed (for reaction and equation, refer the assay of magnesium sulphate under Theory - Chapter 4). Strong ammonia-ammonium chloride solution is used as the buffer so that the pH may be raised to more than 10 and maintained at that level. This is because complexation of magnesium by E.D.T.A. can take place only at this pH. Mordant black is used as the indicator. Appearance of a deep blue colour is the end point.

Procedure: Weigh accurately about 0.3 g of the sample and dissolve in 50 ml of water in a clean conical flask. Add 10 ml of strong ammonia-ammonium chloride solution. Titrate with M/20 disodium ethylenediaminetetraacetate, using mordant black II mixture as indicator till a deep blue colour appears. Each ml of M/20 disodium ethylenediaminetetraacetate is equivalent to 0.00602 g of $MgSO_4$.

Calculation

$$\% \text{ w/w of } MgSO_4 = \frac{T \times N \times 0.00602 \times 100}{\text{Weight taken}}$$

Calculation of Factor

Molecular weight of anhydrous magnesium sulphate = 120.4

$$120.4 \text{ g} \longrightarrow 1000 \text{ ml} \longrightarrow \frac{M}{1}$$

$$12.04 \text{ g} \longrightarrow 1000 \text{ ml} \longrightarrow \frac{M}{10}$$

$$6.02 \text{ g} \longrightarrow 1000 \text{ ml} \longrightarrow \frac{M}{20}$$

$$0.00602 \text{ g} \longrightarrow 1 \text{ ml} \longrightarrow \frac{M}{20}$$

Assay of Magnesium Sulphate Solution

Aim: To assay the given solution of magnesium sulphate and calculate the percentage weight by volume of magnesium sulphate in the solution (% w/v).

Principle: Same as for assay of magnesium sulphate.

Procedure: Pipette out 20 ml of the given magnesium sulphate solution into a clean conical flask. Add 10 ml of strong ammonia-ammonium chloride solution. Titrate with M/20 disodium ethylenediaminetetra-acetate, using mordant black II mixture as indicator until the appearance of blue colour. Repeat the titration to get concordant values. Each ml of M/20 disodium ethylenediaminetetraacetate is equivalent to 0.00602g of $MgSO_4$.

Calculation:

$$\% \text{ w/v of } MgSO_4 = \frac{T \times N \times 0.00602 \times 100}{20}$$

Calculation of Factor:

Same as for assay of magnesium sulphate.

12. Assay of Calcium Gluconate (I.P.1985)

Aim: To assay the given sample of calcium gluconate and calculate its percentage purity.

Principle: An accurately weighed quantity of the sample is dissolved in warm water and 0.05 M magnesium sulphate and strong ammonia-ammonium chloride solution are added. It is titrated against 0.05 M or M/20 E.D.T.A. using mordant black as indicator. Since the change of colour with calcium and mordant black is not very clear at the end point, a known volume of M/20 magensium sulphate solution is added before the titration. The colour change from wine red to blue takes place now distinctly at the end point, when all the calcium and magnesium ions in that order have been complexed by the E.D.T.A. The buffer of strong ammonia-ammonium chloride is added to raise and maintain the pH at 10, because at this pH only complexation takes place. The equivalent of the known volume of M/20 magnesium sulphate in terms of E.D.T.A. is determined by titrating the same volume of M/20 magnesium sulphate separately against E.D.T.A. using mordant black as indicator. The value of this 'blank' titration is deducted from the titre value for both calcium and magnesium in the calculation to arrive at the titre value for calcium alone. For the equation depicting the reaction of complexation of calcium by E.D.T.A., please refer to the assay of calcium gluconate under Theory (Chapter 10).

Procedure: Weigh accurately about 0.5 g of the sample and dissolve in 50 ml of warm water. Add 5 ml of M/20 magnesium sulphate and 10 ml of strong ammonia-ammonium chloride solution. Titrate against M/20 disodium ethylenediaminetetraacetate using mordant black II mixture as indicator. Carry out another titration with E.D.T.A., this time using the same volume (5 ml) of M/20 magnesium sulphate that was used in the first titration and adding the buffer and indicator. Deduct this titre value from the titre value first obtained. (For the purpose of these titrations the M/20 magnesium sulphate solution may be only approximately prepared). The end point in both the titrations is the appearance of a deep blue colour. Each ml of M/20 disodium edetate (after the deduction of the equivalent of M/20 magnesium sulphate used) is equivalent to 0.022420 g of $C_{12}H_{22}CaO_{14}$,H_2O (calcium gluconate).

Calculation

$$\% \text{ w/v of calcium gluconate} = \frac{(T - x) \times N \times 0.022420 \times 100}{\text{Weight taken}}$$

x = Titre value of magnesium sulphate titration

T = Titre value of calcium + magnesium titration.

N = Normality of M/20 E.D.T.A.

Calculation of Factor

Molecular weight of calcium gluconate = 448.40

$$448.4 \text{ g} \longrightarrow 1000 \text{ ml} \longrightarrow \frac{M}{1}$$

$$44.84 \text{ g} \longrightarrow 1000 \text{ ml} \longrightarrow \frac{M}{10}$$

$$22.42 \text{ g} \longrightarrow 1000 \text{ ml} \longrightarrow \frac{M}{20}$$

$$0.02242 \text{ g} \longrightarrow 1 \text{ ml} \longrightarrow \frac{M}{20}$$

Assay of Calcium Gluconate Solution

Aim: To assay the given solution of calcium gluconate and calculate the percentage weight by volume of calcium gluconate in the solution (% w/v).

Principle: Refer assay of calcium gluconate.

Procedure: Pipette out 20 ml of the given calcium gluconate solution into a clean conical flask. Add 5 ml of M/20 magnesium sulphate solution and 10 ml of strong ammonia-ammonium chloride solution. Titrate against M/20 disodium ethylenediaminetetraacetate using mordant black II mixture as indicator. Carry out another titration against M/20 disodium ethylenediamine tetraacetate using 5 ml of M/20 magnesium sulphate solution only. Add the buffer and the indicator before the titration. Appearance of blue colour is the end point in both the titrations. Deduct the titre value of the second titration from the titre value of the first titration. Each ml of M/20 disodium edetate is equivalent to 0.022420 g $C_{12}H_{22}CaO_{14}$,H_2O (calcium gluconate).

Calculation:

$$\% \text{ w/v of calcium gluconate} = \frac{(T-x) \times N \times 0.022420 \times 100}{20}$$

T = Titre value of calcium + magnesium titration.

x = Titre value of magnesium sulphate titration.

N = Normality of M/20 E.D.T.A.

Calculation of Factor: Refer assay of calcium gluconate.

CHAPTER 17

SOME HINTS ON PRACTICAL WORK AND RECORDING

1. WEIGHING

(a) **Chemical Balance:** In the chemical balance there is a central vertical pillar on which rests a horizonal beam. The beam rests on the pillar on an agate knife edge. Similarly at either end of the beam are two agate knife edges on which two suspensions are placed. The two agate knife edges are at the same distance from the central knife edge. One pan each is suspended on each suspension. There is a long pointer attached to centre of the beam and it moves over a scale at the foot of the pillar. This is controlled by a key at the bottom. When this is moved to the left, the beam is released and it oscillates which is shown by the pointer moving over the scale on either side. There are adjusting screws provided on either end of the beam and they can be adjusted for getting the equilibrium position shown by the pointer oscillating to equal distance on either side of the scale.

(b) **Use of Rider:** The beam is divided into 10 main divisions on either side from the centre. Each main division is further subdivided into 5 subdivisions. A rider is a piece of metallic wire shaped in such a way that it can be placed over the serrated beam. Usually the right side of the beam is selected for the use of the rider. By the use of the rider we can weigh anything upto the 3rd and 4th decimals. Each main division is equal to 0.001 gram. Each subdivision lying between the main divisions is equal to 0.0002 gram. Thus while weighing a substance, if the rider is found to be placed at the third subdivision between the fourth and the fifth main divisions, the weight due to the rider is 0.0046 gram.

(c) **Actual Weighing:** First the beam is released and the equilibrium position is got by adjusting if necessary with the adjusting screws. The equilibrium position is indicated by the pointer swinging freely and easily to an equal distance on either side of the zero of the scale. Arrest the beam. The balance is now ready for weighing.

Weighing by difference: Take the approximate weight of the substance in a weighing bottle. Open the left side door of the balance and place the weighing bottle on the left pan. Close the left side door and open the right side door. Place the weights on the right pan. Release the beam and add or remove weights so that equal oscillations are got. Use the rider if necessary.

Then transfer the substance into the appropriate flask or vessel. Weigh the empty bottle again with any substance sticking to it.

Weight of the substance + weighing bottle $=$ a grams

Weight of weighing bottle $=$ b grams

Weight of the susbtance $=$ (a - b) grams.

Weighing by addition: In this tared (previously weighed empty) weighing bottle is used. It is placed on the right pan. The accurate weight (weight of the substance to be taken + weight of the empty weighing bottle) is placed on the left pan. The substance is added in small quantities to the weighing bottle till the correct weight has been added. It is transferred to a suitable flask or other vessel and all the substance sticking to the inside of the bottle is washed with distilled water into the flask or vessel.

2. PIPETTING

A pipette is a narrow long tube tapering to a nozzle at the lower end and with a rectangular bulb in the middle. There is a mark above the bulb. Pipettes are available in various sizes with capacities of 1 ml, 2 ml, 5 ml, 10 ml, 20 ml, 25 ml, 50 ml and 100 ml. Thus a pipette can be used for measuirng *accurately* a particular volume of the liquid and transferring the same to a vessel. For this purpose the lower end of the pipette is immersed in the liquid or solution which is sucked up through the upper end. The liquid is sucked up initially to a level above the mark and closing the top end of the pipette with the middle finger and slowly opening, the liquid is allowed to come down to the level of the mark. Then holding the top end firmly closed, the lower end of the pipette is put into the vessel and the liquid is allowed to drain into the vessel by removing the middle finger from the upper end. After the liquid has drained into the vessel, the last drop remaining in the lower end of the pipette is not disturbed in any way but is allowed to remain in the pipette itself, since the pipette has been calibrated excluding the residual drop.

The pipette should always be cleaned with distilled water and rinsed with the solution to be pipetted out before it is used for pipetting out the solution.

There are two types of pipettes. The pipettes described above are used to deliver a definite volume and are known as volumetric pipettes. The other type of pipette known as graduated pipette is graduated upto a particular length of the tube and can be used to deliver any definite volume within the highest volume marked.

3. USING THE BURETTE

50 ml burettes with stop cocks are commonly used for analytical work. The burette is cleaned with water and fixed in a vertical position in a burette stand. It is filled with distilled water to about 25 per cent of its capacity and rinsed well. The distilled water is then drained out by opening the stop cock. Then about 10 to 15 ml of the titrant is added to the burette, rinsed well and drained out. The burette is then filled with the titrant and the level of the liquid is adjusted to zero. There are one upper meniscus and one lower meniscus in the case of many liquids. The zero may be adjusted to correspond to the lower or upper meniscus. However after the titration is over, the titre value is read off using the same meniscus which was used for adjusting to zero.

4. TITRATION

After adjusting to zero, the titration is commenced by slowly opening the stop cock of the burette and allowing the titrant to fall in drops into the conical flask containing the solution to be titrated and an indicator if necessary and any other substance as prescribed . The titration is done by adding 1 or 0.5 ml initially for each increment but in drops when the end point is nearing. When the end point is almost reached, the stop cock is closed and the titration is stopped. The burette tip is washed with a little distilled water from the wash bottle into the conical flask. It is likely that the end point may now be reached.

For taking down the titre value, the burette is taken off from the burette stand, the level of the titrant in the burette is kept at eye level and the reading is taken. As earlier stated, the reading should be taken at the same meniscus which was used for adjusting to zero.

The conical flask containing the liquid to be titrated is kept on a white tile during the titration so that the end point marked by a colour change or appearance or disappearance of colour may be clearly visible.

5. RECORDING

All exercises done during the academic year should be recorded in a record note book as given below:

On the right page of the record

The title of the exercise is written at the top. At the left hand top corner should be written the Exer. No. and Date. Then the details of the exercise should be given under the following headings:

> Aim
> Principle
> Procedure

On the left page of the record

All the data and the calculations including the calculation for the factor should be written on the left page of the record.

In the case of a titration, the initial reading, final reading and titre value should be given in columns. At the top of the tabular column should be indicated the reactants in the titration. First the substance in the conical flask being titrated is given followed by the titrant. An example is given below:

Oxalic acid x Potassium Permanganate

Oxalic acid solution taken = 20 ml

Initial reading (ml)	Final reading (ml)	Titre Value (ml)
0	21.3	21.3
0	21.2	21.2
0	21.2	21.2

Titre value = 21.2 ml

CHAPTER 18

MODEL QUESTION PAPER - THEORY

Time - Three hours
(Maximum marks : 80)

[Note: (1) Answer Part I and Part II in SEPARATE answer books.

(2) Answer ANY FOUR questions from each part.

(3) ALL questions carry EQUAL marks.

(4) Furnish EQUATIONS wherever necessary.]

PART I   Marks

I. Enumerate the antioxidants used in pharmaceutical practice along with their structures. Discuss the preparation, physical and chemical properties and storage condition of any one of them.   **10**

II. (a) Give at least two methods of preparation of hydrogen peroxide.   **4**

(b) What are the differences in the tests for identity of bicarbonates and carbonates?   **3**

(c) How is yellow mercuric oxide assayed? Give the principle of the assay.   **3**

III. What happens when --   **5 × 2**

(a) sodium thiosulphate is added to iodine solution?

(b) a hot concentrated solution of potassium sulphate is added to a hot solution of an equal quantity of aluminium sulphate?

(c) hydrogen peroxide solution is added to acidified potassium permanganate solution?

(d) a mixture of sodium nitrate and ammonium sulphate is strongly heated?

(e) dilute nitric acid and silver nitrate solution are added to potassium iodide solution?

IV. Give the stability and storage conditions of the following:- 10×1

   (a) Hydrochloric acid

   (b) Potassium acetate

   (c) Sodium fluoride

   (d) Bismuth subcarbonate

   (e) Borax

   (f) Hydrogen peroxide

   (g) Bleaching powder

   (h) Oxygen

   (i) Heavy magnesium oxide

   (j) Sodium hydroxide

V. Write short notes on:-

   (a) Combinations of antacids   4

   (b) Silicone polymers   3

   (c) Combinations of oral electrolyte powders   3

PART II

VI. Discuss the theory of electrolyte balance in the body and give an account of the electrolyte solutions used to restore electrolyte balance.   10

VII. Give an account of the chemical incompatibility in the case of the following substances:

   (a) Bismuth subcarbonate

   (b) Hydrochloric acid

   (c) Magnesium sulphate

   (d) Borax

   (e) Potassium iodide 5×2

VIII (a) Discuss the principle of and procedure for assay of calcium gluconate. **3**

   (b) Give an account of the limit test for iron. **4**

   (c) What is radioactivity? Discuss the detection and measurement of radioactivity. **3**

IX. Give an account of:

   (a) Biological effects of radiation. **3**

   (b) Official buffer solutions. **3**

   (c) Errors in quality control. **4**

X. (a) Outline the principle and procedure for conducting limit test for arsenic. **4**

   (b) Discuss two types of pharmacopial assay for ammonium chloride. **3**

   (c) Give an account of the sources of impurities in pharmacopial substances. **3**